A Little Bit Kinky

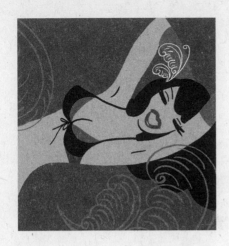

A Little Bit Kinky

A Couples' Guide to Rediscovering the Thrill of Sex

Dr. Natasha Janina Valdez

Broadway Books · New York

BROADWAY

This book is for consenting and informed adults. The author is not a medical doctor, so please consult your physician before trying anything you feel might test your physical limitations. Follow the suggestions in this book at your discretion. The products, positions, and suggestions are safe for the majority of people, but everyone is unique. The author, publisher, and distributors shall have no liability to any person or entity regarding losses or damages caused or alleged to be caused directly or indirectly by the information in this book. Also, please observe the sex laws in your state. We wouldn't want you to get arrested!

Copyright © 2010 by Janina Valdez

Published in the United States by Broadway Books, an imprint of the Crown Publishing Group, a division of Random House, Inc., New York.
www.crownpublishing.com

BROADWAY BOOKS and the Broadway Books colophon are trademarks of Random House, Inc.

Library of Congress Cataloging-in-Publication Data

Valdez, Natasha Janina.
   A little bit kinky: a couples' guide to rediscovering the thrill of
sex / by Dr. Natasha Janina Valdez.—1st ed.
   1. Sex instruction.   2. Sex.   3. Sexual excitement.   I. Title.
HQ31.V227   2010
613.9'6—dc22   2009020439

ISBN 978-0-7679-3244-8

Printed in the United States of America

Design by Lauren Dong

10 9 8 7 6 5 4 3

To my wonderful, loving husband, Charlie Solomon, Jr.,
who consistently teaches me about love, sex, and romance. (Oh, and kink.)

Contents

Introduction 9

Slightly Kinky

1   Romance Is the Rocket Fuel of Sensational Sex 17
2   The Big Tease 33
3   Sexy Places, Sexy People 47

A Little More Kinky . . .

4   Pleasuring Your Partner and Yourself 59
5   I Put My Legs *Where?* 79

Kinkier and Kinkier . . .

6   Tasty, Tantalizing Fun with Food 97
7   Vrrrroom. Whirrrrr. Ahhhh. 115
8   Fun with Fantasy and Role-Play 137

Kinkiest

9   Tie Me Up, Tie You Up 163
10   Lights, Camera, and a Whole Lot of Action 173
11   Sometimes Forbidden Is Fabulous 185

Resources 205
Acknowledgments 207

The word "kinky" probably conjures up all kinds of crazy images in your mind. Leather, whips, chains, and crazy, dangly, medieval devices perhaps? Or risking all kinds of public decency laws? But kinky really isn't that complicated. And it's only as deviant as you want it to be.

"Kinky" is about having fun with sex. It can be as simple as writing your lover's name on your underwear or as wild as making X-rated videos together—and then some. It's about introducing imagination and creativity into sex, about breaking down barriers and savoring true intimacy. Essentially, it's all about breathing new life into your sex life by doing something a little bit different—and, most important, by doing it together.

When you and your partner first got together, no doubt sex was a lot like getting a shiny new toy. Like a kid even weeks after Christmas, you wanted to play with that toy all the time. You pined for it when it wasn't with you, and did everything you could to get it back into your hands.

And there was so much time back then. No kids and countless tasks, no endless activities pulling you in a million directions. If you didn't clean the bathroom or do laundry on a Saturday morning, who cared? Especially if you ditched all these chores because you were snuggled up with that someone special, heavily engaged in countless marathon sessions of mind-blowing passion. And if you've never experienced mind-blowing sex before? Now's the time!

Now, with all you have to contend with, it's easy to see how sex has slipped down the list of priorities and perhaps even right off the radar altogether. But just because you're tired and overextended doesn't mean you need to settle for three-minute missionary sex anytime you're not too wiped out to squeeze it into your schedule. It's time to try something new and to make sex like that fun, new, shiny toy again. It's time to get kinky!

CAN I BE KINKY?

I'm a soccer mom. I'm a partner of a large law firm. I sing at my church. I've been married to the same person for more than twenty years. Can I really *be kinky?*

Of course you can. *Everyone* can be kinky. All that's needed is a willingness, for you and your partner, to explore new possibilities for intimate experiences to share.

It doesn't matter how many thousands of times you've done *it* with your partner; when it comes to sex, there's always something new to discover, a new trick to try. You don't have to take it over the top to make it new again. You just need to be open to all the possibilities there are for you to share.

And that's where *A Little Bit Kinky* comes in. In this book, I'll show you all kinds of ways to push the limits of your inhibitions, to sample and savor new sexual delights, and to learn to communicate and share as a couple better than ever before. And what if you're not in a relationship now—or are just starting a new one—and the sex you've had in past relationships hasn't been that great? Then keep reading to learn how to start your next relationship with the dose of kink it needs.

IS THIS REALLY GOOD FOR MY RELATIONSHIP?

On so many levels, absolutely yes. And you're going to have a great time while you're at it. "Kinky" revitalizes your relationship and solidifies your connection to your significant other, because you just can't pull it off without open communication. And then there's creativity, sensitivity, and a commitment to intimacy. And aren't these exactly the ingredients needed to make a long-term relationship or marriage work?

A Little Bit Kinky is a manual meant for you and your partner to share. It's not intended for you to sneak off and read in a dark corner while your partner is asleep or otherwise occupied (and then left to wonder how you all of a sudden have all this spicy new sex knowledge, as he or she hopes it isn't because you've been doing some outside experimentation). By going through the suggestions together, you'll not only enjoy some good giggling, but you'll also find an easy, unthreatening way to explore and discuss things that may intrigue you. And since most activities can be done by men and women, I've chosen a random gender for each section just to keep the writing clear and easy to understand. Instead of saying "he" or "she," I may simply say "they." Instead of "him" or "her," simply "them." Instead of "his" or "hers," I'll say "their."

Best of all, you won't find long buzz-killing passages of intense instruction here. I've designed this book keeping "the moment" in mind, and thus broken it up into easily digestible bits. That way, when you hit on a suggestion that sounds like something you want to try—right away—you can easily put down your "research" and head into "field study" without losing your place.

The message is simple: You can make sex fun, exciting, and explosive. It doesn't matter if you've been together five, fifteen, or even forty years. By bringing imagination into the bedroom, allowing time to concentrate on romance, making the effort to focus on and cherish your partner, and devoting yourselves to having an insanely, ridiculously, wonderfully fun, uninhibited time together, you can rejuvenate your relationship—and your quality of life. All it takes is a little patience and a little time, a sense of adventure and an open mind, and a desire to *share* with your partner—lust, love, and laughs.

For more than twenty years, I've been coaching all kinds of people about their sex lives. I've also done extensive research on sex, both in the United States and abroad, where the atmosphere surrounding sexuality is more relaxed and open, such as in Europe. I've even interviewed hundreds of male and female sex workers for how they make sex crazy-good. Along the way, I've picked up plenty of ideas on how to spice up the sex lives of even the most timid, tame couples and individuals with all kinds of kinky tips and tricks. And I'm so excited to be able to share them with you.

I have helped singles and couples; people in long-term relationships and those just starting out; people with no kids; people who have just become parents—even people with ten kids. What I have learned is that even the hottest couples go through cool periods, and an infusion of kink can really get the fires burning again. To that end, I guarantee this book will improve your sex life and make your erotic endeavors the best they've ever been.

Some of what I know I've learned from people I've interviewed, but much comes from my own experiences. A healthy amount of kink has been the cornerstone of coupling in all of my own relationships. On top of that, I've traveled around the world visiting strip clubs, dungeons, sex schools, and adult boutiques. I've even owned an adult boutique. I've met with strippers, sex workers, and more. At the end of the day, some of my best ideas have come from regular people, just like you and me—whether through counseling, or through letters, e-mails, and call-ins when I had my own radio show. And now I share all of this with you.

A LITTLE BIT KINKY . . . AND A WHOLE LOTTA FUN

A Little Bit Kinky will help you reconnect with your lover, renew the passion you couldn't live without at one time in your lives, and rediscover why you fell into lust with this person in the first place. Divided into four sections ("Slightly Kinky"; "A Little More Kinky"; "Kinkier and Kinkier"; and "Kinkiest"), *A Little Bit Kinky* runs the gamut of sexual pleasures there are to experience, covering every topic imaginable.

No matter what your skill, experience, or, well, kink level, you'll discover something fresh and exciting to try with your partner and find your way back into a truly satisfying sex life.

Bring a little kink into your bedroom and you'll bring a ton of bonding (and maybe even some bondage) into your relationship. I'll show you how to get back that "new toy" excitement—and even show you how to use some pretty cool toys. I'll also help you discover all the many ways there are to improve your lust life: from tantalizing teases, to sexual positions you don't need to be a pretzel to master, to using foods to heighten sensuality, to fantasy and role-play, to experimenting with light bondage, to creating—and enjoying—visuals, all the way into the most exotic-erotic realm, where only the most adventurous need enter. I've also provided an extensive resource section to show you how to discreetly obtain all the lotions, potions, visuals, props, and notions suggested in each of the chapters.

So get ready to reignite, or ignite for the first time, the fire, passion, and intimacy in your bedroom—and have a hilariously great time while you're at it.

—*Dr. Natasha*
March 2009

Slightly Kinky

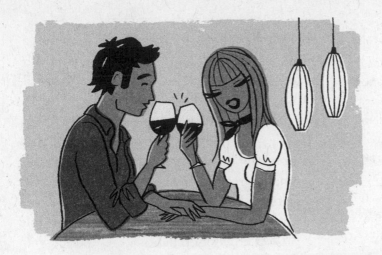

Romance Is the Rocket Fuel of Sensational Sex

Who hasn't complained that since they got married, they just don't ever do it? Or if they do, that it just isn't that much fun anymore? And how many of us swore this would never happen to us when we were dating?

Sadly, most married people don't have enough quality sex. Sooner or later, all long-term couples can fall into a sex rut, especially when you have kids. Parenthood takes a toll physically, mentally, and emotionally. With all the running around and huge expenses adding up, it's easy to see how sex can slip off the list of priorities for both partners. Sex doesn't have to be first on that list for a healthy relationship, but it needs to be pretty high up there.

So let's start at the beginning.

One of the most important ingredients of fun, kinky sex doesn't really have that much to do with sex at all. The first step is to fall back in love, and lust will soon follow. You'll see that if you lay the groundwork correctly, things will start clicking into place. In this short chapter, we'll get reacquainted with the simple art of romance—of showing your partner they are more to you than the one who brings home the paycheck or drops the kids off at school. That they are a person you are still attracted to and want to be closer to.

You may be shocked that something as simple as paying more attention to each other will lead to better sex, and the same goes for doing the dishes when it isn't your night, or complimenting your partner on something they have done well, instead of using all your together time criticizing each other for the things you aren't doing. All of this will rev up the passion between the sheets.

A little romance goes a long way, and it all starts by reminding your partner why you got together with them in the first place. It's possible to help your partner feel like a vibrant, sexual being again and get the satisfaction you crave—without pressuring them into having sex with you. It's all about getting back into the right frame of mind, of helping your partner see themselves as a sexual being again—not just as a parent, employee, roommate, or any of the many roles we play that take our minds far away from sex.

Getting started is easier than you think. It's all about making thoughtful gestures to help you get back in the frame of mind that your relationship is about so much more than keeping your household solvent and your children safe.

LET ME LIST THE WAYS...

A lot of men say their wives or girlfriends complain that they don't get enough romance, but a man's idea of romance can be quite different from a woman's. That's why communication is so very important. When you are direct and tell your partner precisely what you want, when your partner is direct with you and tells you exactly what he or she wants, it cuts out so much wasted time in guesswork and gives you so much more time to actually do what makes the other person happy.

Sometimes it's not easy to ask for things out loud—and you don't have to. Instead, write down on paper what you consider to be a romantic date, and leave nothing to the imagination. Include everything you find romantic, from having the door held open for you to dining in a particular restaurant. Be very detailed from the beginning of the date to the end. Then hand your partner the note and tell him or her that you're craving a little more of this. So many people make the mistake of thinking: "Oh, but if he loves me, *he should just know* what I want." But the only way to ever be sure is to tell him.

Naughty Nibble
Have a T-shirt made that reads "I'm dying to ML2U"—make love to you. It's just another creative way to let your partner know just how much you want him or her.

THE "WE" SPOT

Everyone knows about the G-spot, and no self-respecting sex book should be without mention of it (we'll get to it a bit later). But the only way to get the most satisfaction from the G-spot, and all of the other pleasure centers, is to go through the "We-spot" first.

The We-spot can be a state of mind. We talked about connection earlier—and that's what it's all about. Feel emotionally connected to each other and you'll want to physically connect to each other. Over and over again.

The We-spot can also be a place. Remember when you were in high school and you would need to sneak around to find a secluded spot to mess around, as home was just not an option? Even the thought of that spot way back when was enough to get your fires burning. It was secret, it was sexy, and it was all yours.

So who says you can't have that again? Why not pick a super-romantic make-out place—a lookout point, a baseball field, a beach, a park—anywhere you can take some time out together and talk, watch the sunset, or even make out a little. You can use this spot to celebrate the good times and work through the bad. The important thing is that it's private, that no one else knows where it is, and that it's all yours.

THE LOOK OF LOVE

How much time do you spend looking at your partner these days—I mean really looking at him or her? When you were first in love, you probably couldn't tear your eyes away— perhaps even ogling pictures of your significant other when he or she wasn't by your side. But what about lately?

Staring is an effective, and not to mention hilarious, way to connect with your partner. It forces you to focus your attention on the one all-important place—your partner's face. When I stare at my partner's face I focus on features I already love, notice things I may not have seen before, and develop a deep appreciation for his dimples, his extraordinary eyes. And when I do, I feel closer to him. It's a bonding thing. It's also jarring, in a very pleasant way, for the other person, who's not used to all the attention.

And you can even take it to the next level and make a game of it. Why not have a stare-off contest? Whoever wins gets a kiss, and the game gets hotter as it progresses. It's a silly game that can bring you hours of laughter, not to mention lots of sex if you're good at it. So be sure not to stop at one round. The more you play, the more you'll be collecting—or giving, which is just as good.

Just for Him . . .

There are thousands of ways to show your partner how much you think about her and how much she means to you. Here's one guaranteed to make her feel special—and give her a good laugh: Take a Sharpie and write "I love you, [her name]" across the front of your boxers. Of course, you can get much more graphic than that if you choose to. Whatever you do, just keep the message loving and sexy.

TOWEL, PLEASE

In romance, it's the little things that mean everything, and the most ordinary situations sometimes provide the best opportunities for showing just how much you care. Here's one that fits that bill nicely. The next time your partner takes a shower, plan to be waiting just outside the door for him or her to emerge with a fresh, warm towel you pulled straight from the dryer. And don't just hand it off and leave: Dry them off. Tell your partner with each inch you rub dry how much you love that part—and why. By doing so, you let your partner know that not only are you paying attention to all of him, and that you love and cherish every wonderful inch of him, but that you love to pamper him because he is that special to you.

LIGHTEN THE LOAD

Who doesn't want their life to be a little easier? Is there anything you can do to lighten your partner's load and give her a little more time to herself? Maybe it's something that will help her be more organized, like cleaning out her closet or tidying her drawers. Maybe it's more involved than that. If it usually falls to your partner to clean out the litter box, you do it this time. If you see a laundry basket with clean clothes that your partner hasn't gotten around to folding, get in there and fold. Take his car to the car wash or make the kids breakfast. Doing chores that aren't typically yours not only helps out your partner, but also makes your life more interesting when you aren't doing all the same things. And who knows, your generosity of time and spirit could lead your partner to want to do some of your menial tasks . . . or even return the favor with one of a sexual nature.

BREAKFAST NOOK(Y)

With all the rushing around you do every day, can you even remember the last time you sat down to breakfast with your partner? Now how about the last time it was just the two of you? It seems so basic—to just wake up a half hour earlier to enjoy some quiet alone time—and yet we still choose to hit the snooze button. But it's time to make time, even for just one morning a week. And maybe only one of you gets out of bed to get breakfast ready and treats the other to a few extra minutes of sleep. If it's your day, think of clever ways to add romance to the meal. For example, if you make him oatmeal, arrange raisins into letters on top that say "I love you," "You are special," or some sweet message that will make your partner feel appreciated. Or, if you're feeling frisky, add a dose of kink and spell out "Goddess," "Tie me up," or "I am your slave."

IN THE PARK

When the weather is just right, suggest a picnic. Pack a lunch that you can feed to him with your fingers and take a nice bottle of wine, and be sure to bring along some comfy pillows and a couple of blankets. Lay out the first blanket and put out your spread. Savor feeding each other and sipping the wine and just relax. Place the second blanket over your laps—and let the kink begin. Now stroke each other under the second blanket just enough to get each other going—and without getting caught.

WALKIE, TALKIE

Walking is a great way to get exercise. It's also a fantastic opportunity to connect with your partner by giving you time to talk to each other as you burn off calories. If you don't have kids, or if you have a sitter, take advantage of the half hour after dinner when normally you'd sit on the couch and let your meal collect in fat pockets all over your body. Get up, get moving, and take a thirty-minute stroll instead. And not with your separate iPods. For the first ten minutes, or "the

Work It Off—Work It Up

Exercise helps keep you in shape, but it also has lots of other plusses. Not only does it get your blood pumping, it releases those endorphins that feel oh-so-good. As you work out, you increase your energy level while you improve your blood flow to your genitals, which translates to a higher libido, higher levels of sex hormones, and greater sexual endurance due to an increase in muscle mass. Be active in the following ways at least three times a week for forty to sixty minutes at a time, and you'll not only look good, you'll feel more sexy:

- running
- skiing
- biking
- swimming
- fast walking
- yoga
- jumping rope
- and, the best exercise of all—SEX

Better body, better outlook, better sex. . . . What are you waiting for?

warm-up," go ahead and share gripes from the day. And by that I mean share. Don't take the whole time to complain about your life. Accept that you have your issues to contend with, but that your partner does as well. So listen when it's not your turn to speak.

For the next ten minutes, see if you can offer your partner solutions—any advice that shows you've been listening and want to help. And ask your partner for a solution to your problems. Show them you need them and that their opinion matters. For the last ten minutes, don't talk about anything that bugs you at all. Focus on something that makes you both happy that you're both looking forward to—like planning a vacation or where you might go on your next date night. Or just enjoy the silence and each other's company. Walk with your arms entwined. Or hold hands and reflect on how much you love your partner and how connected you feel to him or her at this very moment. And when you get home, why not top off the trip with a long, passionate, wet kiss?

Just for Him . . .

One hundred percent of women who come to me for therapy tell me their partners don't listen to them. You'd be surprised how happy they become when you can repeat something they've said. So, guys, open your ears and your mouths and let her know, let her *really* know, that you heard her.

GIFT OF LOVE

You don't have to wait for a birthday or anniversary to buy your lover a present. Even if money is tight right now, there's always something that will make him feel appreciated and that you can afford. Be sure to wrap it up nice and attach a note that says something like, "I love you so much and in this box is something you want. But you cannot open it until after we make love." It's an inventive way to come on to your partner, especially if it's been awhile.

Gifts for her could be a love poem or letter, a spa or salon gift certificate, jewelry, a housekeeper, even a coupon book of sexual favors. For him, also a coupon book of sexual favors, as well as a mug for his beer, a special remote control. If you think hard enough about it, you know what your partner likes. But you don't need to guess what these gifts will be. Make this activity easier by each of you making a list of things you'd love to receive and exchanging those lists.

Just for Him . . .

Give your partner a shoulder massage while she's reading or watching TV. It doesn't have to get that involved; it's just a simple, small gesture to show that you care—and that you like to put your hands on her. As an added special touch, rub her favorite scented lotion into her skin and take your time. When you're done, kiss her softly on the nape of her neck and whisper in her ear how much she means to you. And that's it. If she decides to take it to the next level, great. If not, great. The whole point is to be intimate with her without being directly sexual.

TAKE ONE FOR THE "TEAM"

If your partner is a big team sports fan and spends more time on a Sunday in front of the TV instead of with you, don't get annoyed: Work with it. Send the kids somewhere else for the day and plan to spend some sexy sports time with your man. Sit down with him for the game and enjoy it with him. Throw back a couple of beers, ask him questions about what's going on during the various plays. Even if you couldn't care less, feign interest. Make the game something you can share. And then, perhaps at halftime, change the rules and initiate a game of your own. . . .

Now pretend you're no longer in your living room, you're experiencing the game in a strip club. Dress in provocative lingerie and pretend like you're a stripper/waitress. Seductively take his order and bring him beers and snacks on a tray. He can tip you, but he's not allowed to touch you until the end of the game. To keep things really interesting, make several lingerie changes over the course of the game. By the end, even if his team lost, he has another opportunity to be part of your winning team. Now not only have you transformed something that usually annoys you into something kinky, you've shared something with your partner that's important to him—and that will only bring you closer.

SCRATCH MY BACK, I'LL SCRATCH YOURS

Not all your intimate moments need to lead to sex—at least not right away. They can also promote intimacy and heighten your expression of love for your partner. Sometimes it's nice to merely lie together naked and scratch each other's backs. Experiment with different pressures. Lightly scratch, then a little harder. Scratch in long lines the length of her body, then switch to scratching in circles. We'll get into the sexual component of scratching a bit later.

LIKES AND DISLIKES

Everyone has desires and aversions when it comes to sex, and your partner should know them cold. If not, it's time to share. The next time you sit down for a meal together, have two pens and two pieces of paper handy. Hand your partner one of the pens and sheets and suggest he or she write down three things he'd like to try with you sexually tonight—and you do the same. There might be suggestions on his list that you aren't completely comfortable with, but perhaps with a little creative thinking, you can come up with a satisfying compromise. Whatever you do, don't be offended by what you see on your partner's list and don't lose that wonderful playful attitude about the whole process. If you react in any way horrified or repulsed, it will likely shut off your partner to future sexual communication. And that's the last thing you want. If your partner is

> **Naughty Nibble**
>
> Make a list of all the things you love and adore about your honey. When finished, give it to your partner and say: "This is how many times I want to make love to you this week, and these are all the reasons why."

List Mania

Tell your partner that he or she has ten minutes to answer these questions about you—and then you answer them about him or her:

Favorite color? _____

Number? _____

Sexual position? _____

Closest friend? _____

Ice cream? _____

Perfume or cologne? _____

Song? _____

Movie? _____

Vacation spot? _____

Foreplay technique? _____

Place to be touched? _____

Place to be licked? _____

Place to be kissed? _____

Place to be stroked? _____

Sexual fantasy? _____

Place to make love? _____

Time of day to make love? _____

How did he or she do? What does he or she need to learn? How did you do? In what ways should you pay more attention to your partner? It's all about sharing and caring.

horrified, put their fears to rest. Assure them that everything is negotiable, and if they are not comfortable with an idea on your list, calmly suggest you skip it and move on to the next one. Or open a discussion of why your partner is horrified by your suggestion and see if you can't modify it in a way that pleases you both.

JUST YOUR TYPE

Send four erotic e-mails to your lover throughout the day, ranging from mild to wild. The first might read something to the effect of "I've been thinking of you from the minute I woke up this morning" right on to "As soon as you come home, I am going to fulfill your every sexual desire." Make the epistles as erotic as you like—talking about licking and sucking and teasing and touching. By the time he walks in the door, it won't matter what a hard day he had at work, as he'll be oh-so-hard for you. So don't let him down.

> ## Naughty Nibble
>
> Start a pillow fight with your lover tonight. You'll relieve tension and aggression while you bounce around on the bed and get geared up for more. . . .

BRING ME FLOWERS . . .

Pick up a dozen roses for your honey tonight. When you get home, slip one out of the bouquet and tell her to get naked and lie down on her back. When she does, blindfold her with a silk scarf and trace lines all over her body with the petals. Next, pluck off the petals and place them lightly on her body—her belly button, her nipples, wherever your heart desires. What happens next is up to her, but if she doesn't want sex right this minute, don't force the issue. Just lie together and enjoy the moment.

YOU BETCHA

At lunch or dinner today, make a bet about something—a sporting event, the weather, what one of your kids will say next—with the winner being granted a mutually agreed upon sexual favor. It could be one hour of being a sex slave, a full-body massage, or even an oral favor. It's entirely up to you.

EROTIC EXPOSURE

One afternoon when you have a hundred boring errands to get through together, make things a bit more interesting by taking a camera along with you. All day long, snap photos of each other, even while doing something as inane as picking up the dry cleaning or standing on line at the post office, just to show how interested you are in each other. Focus on each other and on your time together—which is what's the important thing in all of this. Compliment each other as you go, letting him know how his eyes sparkle when he reviews the chips options in the grocery store, or how the lighting at the butcher really flatters her. Keep the compliments flowing and snap, snap, snap away.

Later, when you download the pictures or have them developed, they will remind you of how much your partner adores you—even under the most ridiculous circumstances. This may not be the dirtiest way to use your camera, but you'll be laying some serious

Just for Him . . .

Ask your partner out on a date and plan all the arrangements—from where you'll eat and at what time, to what you will actually order. You drive; you pay. After you've had a nice dinner and just before the dessert arrives, slide her a package wrapped up like a birthday gift. In this package will be a sexy pair of undies with a note attached, bearing one simple message: "I'd like to see you in these." Then see if you make it through dessert. . . .

foundation for future friskiness—and look really innocent while you're at it.

BRUSHING UP ON THINGS . . .

Here's something I learned in a spa that you can use to heighten your lover's senses while rediscovering his or her body. Take a dry bristle brush and use it to "brush" your partner. It sounds weird, but it actually feels really good. You can use it to slough off the dead skin, clear pores, and stimulate their body as they start to feel softer and sexier than ever. Brush strokes should always be made toward the heart, starting at the feet and moving up. Skirt around the genitals and use clockwise strokes on the abs. For the grand finale, take a hot shower together and really get that skin tingling.

Just for Her . . .

In a survey of more than five hundred men about what made a woman a great lover, do you know what made the top of the list? Enthusiasm. Men want you to initiate sex more and let them know what you want. So tomorrow morning, why not wake up twenty minutes early and make it obvious that what you want is him.

HOT SPOTTING

This game, which you play naked, teaches you a ton about each other's body. To play, begin touching your lover everywhere—earlobes, nipples, toes, wherever—and have him or her rate how being touched in these places feels on a scale from one to ten. Pay careful attention and repeat touching as necessary. Then it's your partner's turn to explore. The point here is to take an inventory on each other's hot spots—at least once a month, as they are subject to change. Do this and you'll always know just where to touch to keep the passion fresh.

NOW YOU KNOW...

Taking time to step back from life and pay attention to your partner as a person is essential to making them feel like a sexual being again. By doing special things for them, you open the door for all kinds of expressions of love and lust to deluge your relationship.

Now that you've learned how to strengthen your emotional connection, let's move on to the good stuff. In the next chapter, you'll learn all kinds of ways to tease, tantalize, and deliciously torture your lover. Because what's more fun than that?

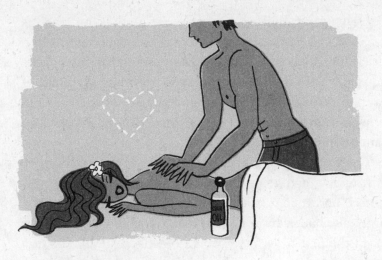

Chapter 2

The Big Tease

When's the last time you and your partner actually took your time having sex? When you made a conscious effort to savor the experience of being naked together rather than just squeezing it into your schedule and "getting it over with"?

Most of us truly can't remember when—and that's not good. Sex is not just a wham-bam-thank-you-ma'am chore, it's a way to get closer and more connected to your partner. And when you draw out the experience, spending more time on actually *experiencing* it and your partner—not just making a mad rush to press all the hot buttons before *The Daily Show* or Leno comes on—sex can take on a whole new dimension. And hey, no one's saying a good quickie can't be fun. Just not every time.

Anticipation is kinky. It's both a power play and a way to show you want to take the time to care. When you tease your partner and prolong the passion, you prolong the pleasure and intensify your orgasms every time.

Don't worry: There's no way we're getting into the ins and outs of Tantric sex or anything like it in this chapter. Please. Who has time to learn and master ancient sex techniques? No, we're keeping it simple, providing examples of ways to have erotic fun without actually doing it—and showing how all this sexy "lead time" will only make you want to do it more.

Teasing is kinky, and there are so many ways to enjoy both teasing and being teased. It's an excellent way to get yourself and your partner so consumed with lust that you'll forget all about why you were too busy to consider having sex in the first place, as all you'll be able to think about is being intimate together. Which is just as it should be.

TEASE APPEAL

Most of the time, married sex starts in bed ten minutes before you go to sleep. But why should it? Of course you have to set careful boundaries if you have kids, but that doesn't mean every event in your sex life has to take place behind your bedroom door. Teasing can be innocent, and many of the ways you can gear up for the big grind hours—even days—before it occurs can take place right out in the open.

A tease can be as simple as slipping a provocative note in your lover's briefcase while you're packing the kids' lunches, or seductively whispering a naughty suggestion into your lover's ear over a sink of dirty dishes. It could be sharing a sexual dream or bringing up a new sexual position in the car on the way to Costco (while the kids are off with friends). Maybe you can't have sex right at these moments, but you can start thinking about it. It's all about showing interest, being creative, and having fun.

FANTASY ISLAND

What could be a bigger tease than sharing a sexual fantasy with your partner when there's no possible way you'll be able to act it out at that moment—or even until much later?

The next time you have ten minutes alone together, forget about discussing which bills need to be paid and what chores need to be done, and exchange sexual fantasies instead. Narrow down your fantasies to your favorites, then agree on one you'll continue to add to verbally throughout the week. For example, if you have a fantasy of making love on the beach, your partner can add to it by saying the sun is going down just as he or she is going down on you. . . . You could add that out of the corner of your eye you see someone watching, and then he or she adds what comes next. Keep it going until the end of the week, then savor your delicious reward when you finally have the chance to act it out.

> ## Just for Her . . .
>
> On your next "date night," present your guy a package wrapped up like a birthday gift. What's inside? A pair of your underwear with a note that reads: "I was wearing these when we left the house."

THE WRITTEN WORD

People have been teasing their lovers with letters since the dawn of time, and it's just as powerful a tool today as it ever was—except now there are all kinds of modern methods to do it.

Here's one way. On an ordinary stack of Post-it notes, scribble out all kinds of sexy messages, naughty and nice:

- I can't wait to come home and be with you.
- I can't wait to come home and kiss you.

- All I can see when I close my eyes is you . . . naked.
- I love your giant . . .

Stick up a bunch of notes at a time, or one a day for several days. Leave them everywhere—on the fridge, on her mirror, on his desk, on her nightstand, on the coffeepot. Just remember: The more provocative the message, the more private the location.

Don't forget about cyberspace. Over the course of a day, send your lover erotic e-mails, each naughtier than the last. The first could say something like "I've been thinking of you all day," and the messages could build to "All I can think about is licking you all over your body" and other, even more explicit messages that pop out of your erotic imagination. Whatever messages you send, just be sure to start off slow and sweet and continue to build.

Naughty Nibble

For a whole day answer everything your partner asks with a direct sexual question, no matter what he or she is talking about. If he says, "Honey, we're out of orange juice," you reply with "What, you want to pour orange juice all over my body and lick it off?" You get the idea. If you keep the game going the entire day, imagine how revved up and ready you'll be when it's actually time to go to bed.

IN OTHER WORDS . . .

If you're not a person of words, not to worry. There's plenty of erotic material out there you and your partner can borrow and have lots of fun exploring. Along with this book, always keep a stash of erotic novels in the top drawer of your nightstand, marking all the racy passages for easy access. If you get a charge out of Victorian erotica, look for a book called *Romance of Lust,* a shockingly sexual coming-of-age novel that was a secret bestseller in its time and was long banned by the preservers of public morality. The next time there's nothing good on TV, turn it off and turn your partner on by reading some of those passages out loud instead.

If you prefer modern erotica, pick up *Penthouse* magazine. Flip through the pages and look for the "Penthouse Forum" section, which contains letters from people detailing some of their craziest sexual experiences. Look through the magazine and choose a favorite letter, then pass it to your partner to give him or her a chance. Once you each hit on ones you like, read them aloud to each other. Just don't touch, cuddle, or have any physical contact with each other while you do. The more you play this game, the more sexual tension you create—and the greater the tension, the sweeter the release.

> ## Naughty Nibble
>
> There's no reason sexplay needs to be fully choreographed down to the climax. Improvisation is most of the fun. So while you can use any of these tips for inspiration, your best bet is to just go with the flow. And don't forget to laugh sometimes. Remember: Sex is supposed to be fun.

SEX BOX

A great way to get your tease on is to create a mystery for your partner, to give him or her something to get curious about. And then, as soon as he or she's ready to explore the possibilities, take it away.

Here's a fun, easy package you can create for your partner. Take an old hatbox or a container around that size and fill it with nothing but erotic objects—perhaps a couple of sexy silky scarves, a vibrator, a scented candle, some lubricant, a sex video. Whatever comes to mind. Then hide the box under the bed or somewhere in your bedroom.

When you want to have a little fun, take out the box and

have him or her reach inside and pull out each of the items. Whatever gets pulled out, explain in graphic detail why it's there and how you plan to use it on your partner. Then put the box away with a sly smile, and leave him or her thinking about its sexy contents for your next erotic adventure.

SURPRISE PACKAGE

As a variation on the Sex Box, put together an erotic surprise package and send it to him somewhere away from home— like at his job. Make sure it includes the following: a pair of sexy underwear with his favorite perfume sprayed on them; a naughty note describing all kinds of sexy things you'd like to do to him; and an erotic photo of yourself—or even a page from the Victoria's Secret catalog, with a picture of your face on one of the models. . . . He'll get a big chuckle out of this one, and so should you. Just be sure to mark the package "Private and Confidential." And get ready for the sexiness it stirs up.

COACH POTATO

At the end of the day, everyone's tired, and not many of us want to get involved in doing anything more ambitious than watching TV. But who says watching TV means no sex? It can if you do it right.

During every commercial break, each of you must remove one article of clothing. When you get to *naked,* that doesn't mean the game is over. Raise the stakes and continue the tease. Now, when a commercial break hits, have your partner point to a spot on his or her body (other than the usual suspects, please), somewhere he or she wants you to touch, kiss, or even lick, and you do just that. But when the show comes back on, stop. Immediately. At the next commercial break, it's your turn to get teased. It doesn't matter how into the program you thought you were; before too long, you'll both be dying for it to end and the real show to begin.

THE CLASSIC STRIP-*TEASE*

This may not be for everyone, but ladies, if you feel brave enough to try it out, you can make your partner absolutely insane with even the simplest routine. And here's where it really gets interesting: Just like a professional exotic dancer, you're going to put on a show for him that he will never forget, but no matter how turned on he becomes, he will not be allowed to touch you and you cannot have sex until morning. Talk about a tease.

Probably the ideal place to set the stage is in your bedroom after the kids are asleep. You don't want anyone walking in on this. You can get fancy, having various props and accessories on hand—a feather boa, a pair of way-high clear heels, a sequined bra and G-string—or you can keep it simple. Yes, props can be fun, but you can still be plenty kinky in your standard button-down shirt and jeans. Just be sure to wear something a little sexy underneath. A ratty old bra or baggy, saggy panties will kill the mood. Also, having some music will not only help you relax, it can also heighten the experience for yourself and for your partner.

Start off slowly and keep that pace. Each action you

Naughty Nibble

Heavy pet tonight on the couch, make out for hours, go to first, second, and third base, but whatever you do, don't do it. I know this makes you out as a big tease, but that's what you're going to be. Resist for at least one hour and watch how explosive the resisting makes your lovemaking.

Just for Her . . .

Here are some of my favorite songs to play with the volume all the way up while you're stripping down:

"You Can Leave Your Hat On," by Joe Cocker
"Private Dancer," by Tina Turner
"Strip for You," by R. Kelly
"U and Dat," by E-40
"Now You're Messing with a Son of a Bitch," by Nazareth
"Welcome to the Jungle," by Guns N' Roses
"Girls, Girls, Girls," by Mötley Crüe
"I Want You to Want Me," by Cheap Trick
"Give It to Me Baby," by Rick James
"Pull Up to the Bumper," by Grace Jones
"Me So Horny," by 2 Live Crew
"I Kissed a Girl," by Katy Perry
"Let Me See the Booty," by The-Dream and Lil Jon
"Shake, Shake, Shake," by KC & the Sunshine Band

perform—unbuttoning each button, pulling down the zipper—should look and feel deliberate to your audience. And most important: Every move you make should be executed while staring your partner square in the eyes. Just remember: No touching till morning.

HIGH AND MIGHTY

Ladies: Pull out your highest heels and wear them around the house with something really skimpy to accompany them. Go find a feather duster and start dusting around the house in your "I'm ready for sex" outfit. If he asks what on earth you are doing, tell him you're feeling frisky today and that you're dying to make love to him with your high heels on. Tell him he has to wait until you're finished with your task before he can pounce—but then he has only one minute to act on your desire. Any more time than that and he'll just have to wait till the next time you feel like you're in the mood.

SMOOCHIN' THE NIGHT AWAY

Kissing can be a very innocent way to express affection, but it can also be a huge tease. Especially when that's all there's going to be. Remember when making out was the only action you got? How you could spend hours with your boy- or girlfriend cuddling and kissing, all the while praying that you could go just a little bit further?

Well, now you can—but sometimes it's nice not to. Bring back that delicious sense of anticipation with your partner with a long, drawn-out make-out session. Go slowly at first, with long, passionate, tongueless kisses. Tease with little pecks, then little bites, and then slowly introduce some tongue action. Show your partner how you like to be kissed by example. You don't want to choke on someone else's tongue, and neither does your lover.

> ### Naughty Nibble
>
> Anyone, including your grandmother, can plant a quick smooch when saying hello or goodbye. You and your partner can do better than that. Each morning and night for a week, plant a twenty-second kiss right on his or her lips. Twenty seconds won't break either of your schedules, but it will boost the anticipation for when you can make that kiss even longer.

Kissing is so incredibly intimate, but couples can sometimes forget how fun it can be, as most of us are always rushing to get to the next step. Just imagine how intense you can each make the experience when there is no next step you're necessarily rushing to.

NAKED YOGA

Did you know that yoga is a natural aphrodisiac? It calms your mind, relaxes the soul, and lightens the spirit. Who wouldn't be ready for making love after all that?

To bring some sexy yoga into your home, buy a DVD, strip down, and begin performing all the various bends and stretches in the raw when you know your partner is about to enter the room. If you have a full-length mirror nearby, even better. Ask your partner to join you, explaining that yoga has been proven to increase blood flow to all areas of the body . . . and is supposed to ignite the libido. Invite your partner to test it out with you and see if you can prove the ancient wisdom—over and over again.

Naughty Nibble

When you prolong the inevitable, the inevitable becomes more exciting. So while furiously tearing away at your lover can be exciting and really charge up both your batteries . . . slowly, torturously stripping items away, piece by piece, can be just as satisfying.

TAKING IT TO THE SHEETS

Just because you're in bed doesn't mean you have to get naked and busy right away. There are so many fun, creative, passionate ways to build a mood and leave your partner and yourself craving more and more.

Here's one kinky pre-bedtime ritual that may appeal only to the most adventurous. Blindfold each other while you're fully dressed. Next, begin to undress each other. As you remove articles of clothing, stroke, kiss, and lick exposed areas. Take your time as you remove the layers, and don't rush to get naked. At no time will you be allowed to take off your blindfolds—even when you're both finally naked. Blindfolded, you'll find your other senses will heighten, and as you take the time to explore each other's bodies without your eyes, it will be all you can do to not tear off your blindfolds and tear into your partner.

SEXY SHAVE

Invite your partner to partake in an intimate shave. Pour baby oil all over your privates and ask him to carefully shave away your pubes, creating an interesting new "toy" to play with later.

Or delight in the element of surprise. Perform the shave yourself and then slide into a pair of your sexiest panties. Later, when you have alone time with your partner, ask him

Just for Him . . .

It's been said that a woman's sexual organs are her brain and her entire body. For that reason, a sexy massage is a great way to get her "in the mood." Not only does the relaxation aspect of it help clear all the clutter out of her brain and start to focus on her body, but the sensation of you touching her all over means she'll be ready to explode when you finally touch her in an overtly sexual way. Just follow these techniques and you'll be well on your way to mind-blowing passion.

1. Make sure she's in a comfy space—on the couch, on the bed— and ask her to undress. Light a candle and make sure to have the massage oils at the ready.
2. Relax her shoulders by kneading them on each side of her shoulder blades. Ask for her input. Does she want more pressure? Does she want less?

3. Work down to her lower back, making small circular motions with your thumbs. When you get to her buns, rub the inside of your forearm in large circular motions on her rear, one cheek at a time. This is what I like to call bun bliss.

4. Instruct her to roll over and kneel by her left side. Gently lift her arm, placing her elbow in your palm. With a light touch from your fingertips, stroke the inside area of her arm. Then take your thumbs and work on the forearms by alternating, pressing in until you get to the hands, and knead the hands with your thumbs alternating. Interlace her fingers with yours and pull back on her palm with your hand, gently now. Give her hand a soft, gentle kiss and do the other side.

5. Rub her legs with long strokes, using the palms of your hands. Alternate between them and push your strokes toward her heart.

6. Move down to her feet. Place a pillow under her knees as she's lying faceup, and with your flat open palms massage the entire foot, slowly and evenly. Move your thumbs in mini circles, then alternate pressing and kneading with your thumbs. (Did you know that feet are a major erogenous zone?)

7. Last, massage her scalp. Take the earlobes in between your thumb and index fingers and rub in little circles, then slide your palms to either side of her head, gently lifting the roots of her hair upward. Lightly scratch her head all over, then with your fingertips lightly massage her temples. Lightly massage her whole head in big circles with your fingertips and finish with the earlobe massage.

After a massage as intense as this, most women will be revved up and ready to go. But don't be too annoyed if you actually relax her so much she falls asleep. She'll make it up to you.

to feel your panties. And then, better yet, ask him to feel under them. . . .

OVER THE EDGE . . . WELL, JUST ABOUT

Sometimes one partner gets so concerned with the other's pleasure, he or she may find it difficult to just sit back and let stuff happen to them. And that's not really any fun.

If you're usually the "submissive" partner, shake things up a little by taking matters into your own hands. Tell your partner it's your turn to call the shots and they are not allowed to move, kiss, lick, or touch you until you say it's okay.

Start out with your partner lying comfortably on his or her tummy. Massage the shoulders, neck, and back. If you have it (and you really should have it), break out the massage oil, warm it in your hands, and really work it into your partner's skin.

Once you feel the tension begin to release, it's time for the front. Massage their legs and feet and even toes. Lightly run your fingers all over your partner's body, and pay attention to the way they respond to your touch. Only graze your partner's most intimate parts. Don't you dare touch them. At least not yet. Hold out for as long as you both can, and enjoy the sensation as the tension builds.

Just for Her . . .

Here's a game you'll enjoy keeping your clothes on for. Put on a skirt but don't put on panties. Now find your man, climb onto his lap, face him, and wrap your legs around his waist. Expose yourself to him as you unzip his pants. Pull out his penis and teasingly play with it. Rub it up against you and, as he starts to get turned on, slip just the tip of his penis into your vagina—then quickly pull it out. Keep repeating the tease, and don't let him enter you fully until he tells you five things he absolutely adores about you. Keep in mind, though, that most of the blood has rushed away from his brain. So if he's a bit slow to answer, just be patient—and enjoy prolonging the passion.

NOW YOU KNOW...

The anticipation of sex can be as delightful as the act—and can really enhance how your partner will respond to all the luscious delights that await. And we'll get into the nitty-gritty of many of these delights in the coming chapters. But first: the setting.

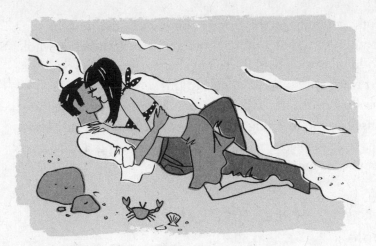

Chapter 3

Sexy Places, Sexy People

t is possible to have hot kinky sex anywhere, including your bed. But when's the last time you had sex in a place aside from your bedroom? Or even outside your house? Think about it for a minute. Not coming up with anything? That's what I thought. That's what it's like for many couples who congratulate themselves for even finding the time to have sex at all. And if they can have hot passionate sex—an even louder round of applause! No one's saying bed sex can't be kinky . . . but the fact of the matter for most of us is that having the sex at all is a stretch. So to think about having it somewhere else, to actually plan for that sort of thing, well, it seems like it would take a miracle.

Guess what? You can make your own miracles. And most of the time, you never even have to leave your own property. (Although sometimes you really should.) Probably you've considered—and even tested out—the erotic potential of the living room couch, the desk in your home office, your dining room table. But there's a whole world of erotic possibilities out there waiting for you if you just reach out and seize them. In this short chapter, I'll show you how to think outside the box when setting a scene for sensuality—reminding you of things you may already know but have managed to forget, and introducing a wealth of brand-new possibilities.

Naughty Nibble

Consider mirroring an entire wall—or even the ceiling—in your bedroom or another more "innocent" room in your home, because watching yourselves do it can be a huge turn-on. And if anyone comments on the mirrors, tell them you read in a magazine that mirrors "open up a space" and "make it seem bigger." (They probably won't make the connection, so the double entendre is yours to enjoy.)

PLEASURE DEN

A sexier environment makes for a sexier life, and for that reason, it's time to revamp your bedroom and make it more conducive to passion. You could go so far as to repaint the walls in a warm tone and hang only the sexiest artwork—or, on a more simple scale, just be sure to keep all ancillary clutter at a minimum. Your night table should not have stacks of bills and school permission slips and other sex killers, but rather votive candles in romantic holders, framed photos of you and your lover—and by this I mean only the ones in which you look your best and in which your kids aren't featured.

Create a romantic atmosphere with silky scarves draped about and perhaps incense close at hand. And your night table drawers should contain items for sexplay: toys and lubricants, lotions and oils, scarves and restraints—whatever you're into.

CARNAL CLOSET

A change of scenery can do wonders for your sex life. But you don't actually ever even have to leave your own house to experience passion in a strange and sexy setting. Just look around.

Is there any place in your home that could be imagined into a sex den? How about the closet? If you have one large enough to accommodate a raucous romp, well, go for it.

Do a little advance planning for this one. Without your partner's knowledge, clear out all the crap crammed into your closet and deck it out instead as a love nest, complete with plenty of pillows and silky soft linens. Grab a flashlight and your lover and bring him or her into your newly converted love nest. Turn out all the lights—and just use the flashlight sparingly. And now get down to it.

OCEANFRONT

If you live close to a beach, there are few pleasures as exotic and erotic as making love in the surf. Of course, if you don't, you can still make some pretty sexy memories with a little creativity and imagination, as you make your own seaside haven in your bedroom.

Invest in a CD of sounds from the ocean and play it softly. Light candles scented with ocean breezes, and be sure to get some scented massage oil or lotion reminiscent of the beach.

Just for Her . . .

Next time you're lying together naked, spark up the candles, light the incense, and tell him to lie back and relax. Run a silky scarf around his neck and all over his body. Wrap another scarf around his penis, starting from the base, until it's completely covered. Now, with your fingernails, lightly graze the skin all over his body.

Just for Her . . .

Plan a trip to the mall on some random night and tell your sweetie he has to come along. If he resists, as he probably will, insist you can make it worth his while.

First off, leave the house wearing nothing but high heels and a raincoat. When you finally make it to the mall, make a beeline for the lingerie store. Stroll around together and browse the offerings. Make some selections, and invite him to choose some skimpy items he'd like to see you in. If you're feeling truly kinky, try to sneak him in to watch you try things on. But if that's too risky for you, make a few select purchases (including pieces he hasn't seen you pick out) and head home for a fashion show he'll never forget.

Invite your partner to your ocean paradise and lead him or her to the bed. Be sure you're wearing your bathing suit; for your partner, it's definitely bathing suit optional. If desired, offer your partner a tropical cocktail and have him or her lie down on tummy or back—whichever is more comfortable—telling your lover that this is all about relaxing.

Now take the massage oil or lotion and treat your honey to a full-body massage as he or she takes in the sounds of the surf and the scents that surround.

If your lover chooses tummy first, have them lie on their tummy, and start by massaging the shoulders, neck, even scalp, and move on down the back. Massage down the back to the tush, giving it a lot of concentrated attention. Rub the oil or lotion into their arms, wrists, hands; thighs, ankles, feet. You can run your hands up and down your partner's sides, even grazing the very edge of his or her special parts. But don't touch those parts—at least not yet.

Now tell your lover to flip over. Massage the face, neck, shoulders again and then down the front to the breasts or pecs and the tummy. Massage around the genitals but, again, do not touch them—not until your partner is begging and squirming, that is. Then open the floodgates and let the wonderful waves of pleasure wash right over you both.

RAISE THE ROOF

Or at least don't forget it's there—and makes a great erotic venue. You probably only want to hang out on the rooftop if you live in an apartment building or if your house has a flat roof, because you don't need to worry about falling while you're soaring to new heights of ecstasy. Decorate your roof with romantic votive candles and soft silky fabrics and pillows, and be sure to have a nice bottle of champagne chilling nearby. Have you ever made love under the stars? It's an experience you'll never forget!

OH, STARRY NIGHT

You don't have to take to the rooftops to savor sensuality in the great outdoors. The next night the stars are bright and there aren't any clouds in the sky, plan an erotic picnic involving foods you can feed each other with your fingers, perhaps a bottle of champagne, a soft blanket to dine on, and not a stitch of clothing between you.

TENT THIS

And if the idea of hanging out together outside is more terrifying than titillating, take it inside—inside a tent, that is. Some tents even have "windows"—holes at the top covered with clear plastic that give you a great view of the stars and make you feel like you're outside, but with much less risk of getting caught.

HANGIN' IN THE HAMMOCK

What could be more relaxing than swinging back and forth in your backyard hammock? If you're relaxing with your honey, why not add a little action? There are plenty of sexual activities to enjoy as you swing back and forth, but the fun part comes in testing how well you can actually balance while you're at it. There may be more laughs than orgasms with this trick, but isn't that part of the fun?

THE HIGH SEAS

If you like the motion of a hammock, set the stakes even higher—with a bawdy boat trip. Sure, you can take a couples cruise and head to your stateroom to get your own boat a-rockin'. But what about taking out a sailboat or motorboat and making love in the middle of the sea? Better yet, how about a romantic rendezvous in a rowboat? Or, if you want to really test your abilities to balance, try a canoe. Just know you're probably going to get very wet. In a good way. And you're going to love every minute of it.

TOURIST TRAP

Make a reservation at the classiest hotel you can think of—or at least afford—and invite your partner to dine in the hotel's restaurant with you that night. As you enjoy your meal, remind your partner to "eat light," as you have it on the best authority that the dessert here is the best in town—a real decadent experience. After dinner, excuse yourself to the powder room and slip away to the front desk to pick up two sets of keys, order some strawberries and champagne for the room, and pay the dinner bill.

When you return, suggest to your partner that he or she go "freshen up" while you wait for the dessert that you pretend to have already ordered. Take this opportunity to put the key at his or her place, then hightail it out of there. Head to the room and strip down to your sexy skin and wait for the room service and your partner to arrive. This dessert is sure to get raves.

Surely you could enact this scenario in your own bedroom, but there's something about being away from home—the privacy, the distance from the kids, the escape from the telephones and everything else that constantly consumes you. And the best part about it is that you can get as wild, loud, and messy as you want!

SNEAK ATTACK

Next time you're at a party, mingle, relax, and enjoy. And then sneak off with your partner to a bedroom, bathroom, coat closet—or wherever you can savor a thin slice of privacy. If you can, lock the door behind you. And even if you can't, get down with some thrilling quickie sex. The "fear" of getting caught will surely slip you into high gear. Then rejoin the party as if nothing ever happened.

THE RIDE OF YOUR LIFE

On your next date night, instead of dropping money on dinner and a show, why not rent a limo instead—and really make a night of it. It doesn't matter where you take the limo.

You don't need a destination. Just enjoy the luxury of it. Pretend that you're a couple of glamorous celebrities on your way to some magical event. Whatever gives you the biggest charge.

Pop open a bottle of ice-cold bubbly and savor the sexy suds as you scheme salaciously. And while you plot and dream, be sure to share those frisky fantasies with each other—and even act them out. Just go wild. After all, that's what that partition between you and the driver is for.

AUTO-EROTIC

The next time you're in the car alone together, put in a sexy CD—perhaps something by Enigma or Madonna's *Erotica*. If you're driving, keep your eyes peeled for a quiet spot to pull over. If your partner's driving, make up some excuse for her or him to pull over. When you're parked, straddle and seduce your partner. Who cares if people can see? That's half the fun.

ROOM WITH A VIEW

It's nice to have a hotel room with a view—and especially nice if there's a balcony from which to enjoy it. Because in addition to being a fun spot to hang out, a balcony is also a great place to get down and dirty with the thrill of having sex outside and in public, but at the same time being secluded and private. You can do it on the floor or on a chaise longue if the balcony has one. You

---

Naughty Nibble

Remember the famous Aerosmith song called "Love in an Elevator"? Now, that's a fun one to act out. The next time you're in an elevator together, make a pass at your partner each time the door closes. Even take it to the next level if you dare, with passion fueled by the threat of the elevator stopping to pick up another passenger at any moment.

can do it standing up, leaning over the rail. Whatever you do, just be careful you don't get too carried away and lose your balance. Good sex is supposed to make you feel like you've died and gone to heaven—but not in a literal sense!

BRANCHING OUT

Is there a tree house in your backyard? If you have kids, chances are there is. Send those kids away for the weekend and enjoy the space for yourselves. Pack an erotic picnic for two (see Chapter 6 for suggestions) and get ready to climb to new sexual heights!

POOL PARTY

They're out of town—again. They've asked you to take in their mail, feed their cat, even drop off some bills at the post office when they're due—again. But they're nice enough neighbors. Every time they go away, they offer you use of their pool. So why not make a night of it? Check on their house tonight, feed those cats, and then head outside with a chilled bottle of champagne, two glasses, and one thing on your mind—that scene in *Showgirls* where Elizabeth Berkley gets pounded in the pool as she thrashes and splashes around.

DEAD SEXY

Scared you with that—didn't I? What I'm talking about here is not nearly as taboo as necrophilia, which is way, way past the line of kinky. No, what I'm talking about here is sex in a cemetery. Certainly this scenario is not for everyone, but if you and your lover have some dark fantasies about ghouls and other creatures of the night, what better place is there than this to act them out?

NOW YOU KNOW...

Sex can be sensational when you break out of the confines of what's considered the "norm," which is what we're doing all over this book. In this chapter, surely the added element of the possibility of getting caught only punches up the kink level. In the next section, we'll explore all kinds of kinky new ways you can spruce up old tricks, and definitely the less normal, the better.

A Little More Kinky

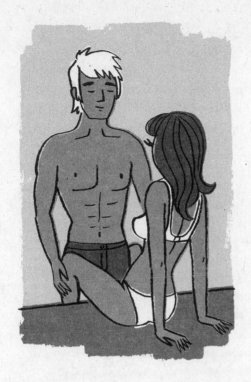

Chapter 4

Pleasuring Your Partner and Yourself

Sex is the way that your relationship with your partner differs from all other relationships in your life. It is the only thing you share exclusively with that person and is the glue that keeps you bonded. So you have to keep "reapplying" it in new and adventurous ways to keep it fresh.

That being said, this book is not a how-to manual for things you've been doing with your partner all these years. I'm not going to give you a beginner's guide in how the clitoris works or how to pleasure a penis. If you've gotten this far in your relationship, chances are pretty good that you know some of these things already. My intention is to show you new twists on the old standards. To provide added tips and tricks you may not be familiar with, and also to show how an imaginative variation goes a long way when it comes to out-of-this-world pleasure.

For some sexual tastes, the act of oral sex may be considered kinky, but for our purposes, that's considered a standard. Same goes for mutual masturbation. What we're going to do here is add a dose of kink into the works and see how daring we can get.

Love Muscles

It's no secret that fit people have more fabulous sex. But did you know there are specific muscles you can exercise that will directly affect your performance and experience in the bedroom? It's true. Your butt and lower abdomen elevate the pelvis and make it easier for you to have close contact with your lover, and inner-thigh muscles can actually compensate for weak vaginal muscles. When in the act, contracting the thighs and butt together can squeeze the penis, giving both partners added pleasure. And strong pelvic floor muscles make for more intense orgasms—and who doesn't want those? Here are three excellent exercises that you can do to strengthen those love muscles. For maximum effect, do at least fifty of each every day.

1. Lie on your back, knees bent, hands behind head, and lift your upper body by crunching up your abdomen.
2. Lie on your back, knees bent, shoulders on floor, and raise just your pelvis off the floor. Hold and squeeze for a count of thirty—or as long as you can hold at first, and work up to thirty—and more.
3. Lie on your back with your legs straight up in the air and held together. Now slowly let them drop to the sides, spreading them as far apart as you can, and slowly pull them back together.

PLEASURE YOU'LL TREASURE

What's good for the goose may be good for the gander in many ways, but when it comes to the mechanics of sex, nothing could be less true. For that reason, I've divided the tips in this chapter into three distinct sections: "What a Girl Wants," "A Man's Desire," and "A Little of This, a Little of That"—for kinky pleasures both can enjoy together. Even though they're divided by gender, I still encourage you to read them together and open the discussion for "I'd like to try that," "I think that feels good," and "If you ever try that on me, I will divorce you."

WHAT A GIRL WANTS...

As we touched on briefly in the last chapter, a woman's main sex organs are not her genitals: They are her mind and her body. So when you approach a woman in a sexual fashion, do not, I repeat, DO NOT hone in on her genitals like a heat-seeking scud missile. You will be spending a lot of time exhausting yourself rubbing and licking as you try to arouse her, when you could accomplish the same feat in minutes—even seconds—by taking the time to pleasure those top two organs first.

> ### Naughty Nibble
> Ladies, is your underwear drawer full of tattered, torn, saggy, and stained underwear? There's nothing kinky about that. It's time to weed through your collection and throw away anything that doesn't make you look and feel absolutely gorgeous. Good-bye sensible cotton briefs; hello silk, lace, and satin thongs.

Mind Yourself

If you haven't already guessed it, the tips in the last two chapters are what you need to use to pleasure her mind.

When she feels valued and appreciated, she feels sexy. When she can anticipate what's to come, she can focus more readily on the act of passion—rather than being ambushed by your amorous actions. Give her a chance to get into the moment, and the moments that follow will be that much more satisfying and rewarding for you both.

Body Beautiful

In the last chapter, we walked through how to give a woman a full-body massage, and we also did some hot-spotting to learn what her erogenous zones may be—which are not always the obvious ones. So before you go lurking around any part of her, revisit what you've already learned and work on those areas first. Light strokes, gentle kisses, hot breath on her skin, a tongue that caresses rather than probing or digging . . . You can amp up the enthusiasm later, but to get started, the name of the game is "soft and slow."

Belly Rub

Here's something not a lot of men know when it comes to pleasuring a woman: Having her belly stroked and rubbed can be very comforting and very stimulating for a woman. With a light touch, and in a clockwise motion, graze her tummy first with your fingertips and escalate to your palms. Focus on the area right below the belly button and right above her pubic hair—but do not touch the pubic region. At least not yet. This not only feels nice for her, it brings the blood flow down to her nether regions, which means her orgasm will be that much more intense and explosive. Are you able to scratch or rub her tummy as you manually stimulate her with your other hand or orally pleasure her? Try it if you can—and maybe she can even lend a hand. It will bring her the orgasm of her life.

Naughty Nipples

For some women, but not all, the nipples are very sensitive to stimulation, and there are so many ways to arouse them. Instead of the usual "grab and squeeze," try using the light touch of the tip of your tongue or blowing on them. A gentle nibble, a luscious lashing . . . Imagine all the ways you could pleasure her with whipped cream, oils, a delicate feather, an ice cube, or hot wax. As you experiment, encourage her to rate each experience from one to ten—with ten being super-fantastic and one being "never, never again."

Peace Out

Here's a good trick to giving her a wholly satisfying erotic massage—and remember, only after you've "awakened" the rest of her. First, apply lots of lube all over her vagina and your fingers. Manually stimulate the area around the tip of her clitoris by rubbing your palm on it in little circles; then switch off to a light fluttering of your fingers; next, make a peace sign with your fingers as you place them on either side of the clitoris and glide them up and down, up and down. With the two middle fingers from your free hand,

Naughty Nibble

A famous actor I know, who also happens to be renowned for his performances in the bedroom, once told me the secret to giving great oral pleasure is to kiss a woman downstairs the way you'd kiss her upstairs.

Naughty Nibble

The U-spot is located at the opening of the urethra, just in front of the vaginal opening. There are a plethora of rich nerve endings here that are ripe for stimulation. Give it a try.

gently slide in and out of her vagina, being sure to pulsate the tips of your fingers on her G-spot. Go back and forth from stimulating her clitoris to her G-spot as she edges closer to orgasm, and repeat the motions until she can't take it anymore.

The Figure 8

Point your tongue and trace figure 8s on her lower region, starting underneath the clitoris and around to the right, over the top of the clitoris, and back where you started. As you make your 8s, make bigger loops every time, finally encompassing the lower lips of the vagina and coming back to underneath the clitoris. Try this slowly and build speed up to her inevitable climax.

The Silky Smooth Three-Eyed Turtle

With massage and light tongue strokes all over her body, work her up so she's on edge and tingling with desire. Now it's time to manually stimulate her clitoris with the head of your penis. Pretend the tip of your penis is an extension of your finger and gently make eight circles around the clitoris to the right, then eight to the left. Pulse upward underneath the clitoris eight times, then push just the tip of your penis into her vagina. Repeat this over and over again, each time giving her just a little more of your penis. She may start begging you to push in your entire member—but don't. The more you prolong her delicious "agony," the more the sexual tension will build in her and the more explosive her orgasm will be.

Rock the Boat

Take your hand and curve it into a C. Lube your thumb and gently insert it into her vagina. Now, with your hand curved like a hook over her pubic bone, rock it back and forth, using your palm to stimulate her clitoris while your thumb stimulates her G-spot and the inside of your hand stimulates her U-spot. To heighten her pleasure past her wildest expectation, now seal it with a kiss. In other words, go down on her, gently dabbing at her clitoris while you continue the rocking motion. Mastering this technique alone will make you a total sex god in her eyes.

Give Her a Hand

After applying lots of lube to your hand and to her area, straighten your hand and with the pinky side rub gently against each side of her inner labia in a sawing motion. Then make a V with the index finger and middle finger on the same hand, and glide up and down on each side of her clitoris. Last, but not least, lube your palm and place it just under the clitoris as you massage the entirety of the vagina in big circles to the right for ten and then to the left for ten, and repeat until she lets you know it's time.

Nympho's Desire

Here's a technique that requires a product called Nympho's Desire. It's enriched arousal

---

Naughty Nibble

Lubricant is everyone's friend. It creates a smooth sensation for her, which heightens her pleasure. For him, it ensures a smooth glide for his penis—wherever it may be gliding. Friction has its place, but too much can be uncomfortable and even painful for both parties. Saliva is a wonderful, easy, and one hundred percent natural lubricant, but there are also many products available. (See Resources.)

Just for Her . . .

Be a Love Teacher and show him how to satisfy you. What are some of the things about sex you really love? Would you like him to suck on your clitoris while he massages your G-spot? Would you like him to nibble your nipples as he thrusts his fingers inside of you? He doesn't know unless you tell him. He's an eager student and wants you to be his teacher. So what are you waiting for?

cream formulated to heighten erogenous zone sensitivity and enhance sexual response. I've used it plenty of times and will forever have a stash in my bedside table—it's guaranteed to make her crazy with lust. With your hand all balmed up, rub gently around her clitoris, then along the lips of her vagina. It will begin to tingle and make her feel hot. Keep massaging her vaginal area with your fingers, as you would massage any other part of the body. As her heat intensifies, so will her orgasm.

G Force

Here's an excellent way for a woman to have a G-spot orgasm. Put a pillow at the base of her spine during intercourse so that her pelvis arches forward as her partner thrusts. The man should imagine that he's aiming for her belly button each time he enters her. With every stroke, she should grab his hand and lightly press her abdomen down with it, which will make the connection with his penis and her G-spot much greater. The woman should let him know what she is feeling, and let him know when she is about to come. She shouldn't be afraid to let go and enjoy her orgasm, as she may have a mounting desire to urinate. It only feels that way—she won't actually urinate—so there's no reason for her not to let go and enjoy the sensation.

Double Trouble

Want to give your lover a truly extraordinary sexual experience? How about a double orgasm? When you manually stimulate your partner, use a soft, slow touch. Move your index finger around and around her clitoris in light circles. When you get to ten, lightly skim the top of the clitoris and reverse the direction for ten more circles. As her excitement builds, slowly glide the index finger of your free hand into her vagina, focusing rubbing the tip of your finger on the upper front wall of her vagina. Go back and forth, stimulating the clitoris and then the G-spot. The desired result is a double orgasm (clitoral and G-spot), but the intensity of the situation may just have her begging you to finish her off with intercourse.

Zee French Tickler

Place both your middle and index fingers inside her vagina and twist your fingers over and over again. You can vary the motion by moving your fingers back and forth in opposite directions very quickly, or add an oral twist as you swirl your tongue around her clitoris at the same time you're performing this maneuver. And *voilà*—orgasm!

The Greatest Show on Earth

There isn't a man on earth who doesn't enjoy watching a woman pleasure herself. The

Naughty Nibble

Have you ever asked your partner to masturbate in front of you? If you'd like to learn what kind of stimulation he or she really gets off from, then this is how you find out, well, firsthand. Also, most men love watching their partners bring themselves to orgasm—yet less than 6 percent of women actually feel comfortable doing so. I think it's time to even out those odds, ladies.

Love Muscles

Do you know that women who Kegel are more orgasmic than women who don't? Kegels are a great way to tighten the vaginal muscles after childbirth—and even make them stronger. Do you know what Kegels are? If you don't, pay attention, because after only a week of Kegel workouts, you'll be having the orgasms of your life.

The next time you're urinating, stop the flow of urine and isolate this muscle. Now you know which muscle you need to strengthen. Now, every day for the next week, squeeze and pulsate this muscle a hundred times a day. Does that seem like a lot? How about twenty squeezes five times a day? That's manageable. After you've done these for a week, ask him to stop moving the next time you have intercourse and squeeze and pulsate the muscles around his penis. This technique alone should revolutionize the way you make love and give you the most pleasure possible from intercourse.

problem is that women get so shy about it. But don't. He wants to see it. He wants to know what makes you feel good. With that in mind, be confident about rocking his world. Start with a subtle suggestion and move into a full-on pleasure fest. Straddle him as you pleasure yourself, and let him see, up close and personal, how your finger lustfully plunges in and out of your vagina; how you rub your clitoris the way you like it and bring yourself over the top. This may be the hardest part of all—but it's the most effective: As you are about to come, look him straight in the eyes and try to keep eye contact as your orgasm washes over you. You'll barely need to touch him to bring him to orgasm after this.

The Sandwich

Here's a real turn-on for when you're going down on her. Take your index finger and thumb and squeeze her vaginal lips together, gently, up by the clitoris. This creates a "sandwich," with the clitoris as the filling. Now place your tongue at the top of the sandwich and lick up and down from the top to the bottom—like you'd lick the cream out of an Oreo cookie. Repeat as desired.

Just for Him . . .

Some surefire techniques for giving her mind-blowing oral sex:

- *Start out right.* Be sure to pull back the clitoral hood so the clitoris is exposed and standing to attention.
- *Lightly at first.* Experiment with the surface of your tongue as you pleasure her. Fold it, flatten it, point it, and swirl it around her clitoris.
- *Turn up the intensity.* Stiffen your tongue and dip it into her vagina every thirty seconds or so.
- *Chill her out.* With an ice cube, drip cold droplets on her clitoris and lick them off.
- *Sound it out.* Move your tongue over her clitoris, pronouncing "tuh-kuh tuh-kuh" over and over again. Then gently suck on her clitoris. Then repeat the "tuh-kuh-tuh-kuh."
- *Breathe heavily.* Exhale deeply as you go down on her and let her savor the sensation of your hot breath—which also feels good on the nipples.
- *Kiss her lovingly.* Kiss her lips down there as you would her lips up there.

Espresso Yourself

Talk about hot oral sex. . . . The thrill of this technique comes from the warmth of the beverage. So if you're not a coffee drinker, by all means substitute hot tea. Keeping the liquid in your mouth:

1. Flatten your tongue and lap around and around her clitoris, counterclockwise, for a count of ten. Swirl the liquid in your mouth, and then swallow or spit out. Keep liquid in your mouth—you want to keep your tongue and mouth hot and moist throughout. Reverse for another count of ten.
2. Now place your middle and index fingers inside her vagina, applying moderate pressure to the G-spot area. Leave your fingers inside her and don't move them around, except to press upward.
3. Lightly suck on her clitoris, placing your whole mouth over it and lightly flicking it with your pointed tongue.
4. Arrange your body so your lips parallel her lips. Pucker your lips and lightly brush your lips to hers back and forth, back and forth. Repeat several times, then stick your tongue out just enough to poke out from your lips and continue until she reaches her climax.

A MAN'S DESIRE

Okay, ladies. So you know how your main sex organs are your brain and your body? Now look at your partner. Can you guess what his are? It's just what you think: his penis and

Just for Her . . .

Call your man at work and ask him to pick up the following items on his way home: baby oil, a razor, and a package of straws. First you'll get him all aroused by asking him to shave you. And then you'll drive him—okay, you—over the edge.

Tell him to grab one of the straws and blow lightly on your clitoris. It will tickle you and feel sensational all at once. Now tell him to place the straw on your clitoris and ask him to lightly suck in pulsating motions. If you like the way it feels, have him continue pulsating the straw by quickly sucking in and out right until you climax. Now, that's kinky. (Note: If he cuts the straws in half first, the sensation of the hot air hitting you there will be much more intense.)

his testicles. This is not to say that a man doesn't enjoy a little stimulation to other parts of his body. Or that his frame of mind has no bearing on his sex drive—because it does. But not nearly to the degree that it does for women. You know how we advised that you can't just head for a woman's genitals and start working them out without prior stimulation to other areas? Not true for a man. But that doesn't mean a little bit of kink isn't going to give him a whole lotta pleasure—as we'll see in the following pages.

Give Him a Hand

A hand job is an old standby: a quick way to get your man off if you're not in the mood. Good hand friction is the name of the game, but that friction needs to be smooth and silky—so first break out the lube and give your hand and his penis a good dousing.

Start with your right hand at the base of the penis, stroke to the top, and then let go. Next, use your left hand and perform the same action, alternating hands about once a second. Vary your speed from fast to slow—but not too slow (he'll let you know). And be sure to use firm pressure. Occasionally, glide your hand over the top of his penis.

While you're manhandling your man, take your other hand and very lightly cup his testicles—just be careful not to squeeze them. This extra bit of stimulation could drive him right over the edge.

Just for Her . . .

Most women hold a man's penis with their knuckles pointing upward, but the underside of the penis is actually the most sensitive part. Next time you're handling your man, switch your grip so that your fingers point down now and the inside of your knuckles stimulate the opposite side.

The Time of His Life

Just for fun, tell your man you want to see how fast you can make him come. Grab the timer from your kitchen or buy a new one to keep in the bedroom and set it for five minutes. Put a wager down. If you get him to come before five minutes, then he has to take you out to dinner to a restaurant of your choice or buy you a pair of shoes you've been eyeing—or even owe you a sexual favor. It's entirely up to you. Just remember that it works both ways, and if he holds out, he gets to claim his own prize.

The GM (Groin Massage)

Want to give your man an erection like never before? Tell him to strip and lie down on his back. Spread his legs about two feet apart and cover his groin in massage oil. Starting on his left side, press your left palm gently into the bottom of his groin and push up toward his heart; alternate with the right hand on his right side as you get a rhythm going. Repeat for fifty strokes to really increase the blood flow to his penis and give him a stronger erection than ever before.

The Best BJ Ever

Here are tips to follow to ensure that the next blow job you give your partner is the one he never forgets.

- *Be enthusiastic.* If you show him you love it, it will be an incredible turn-on for him.
- *No teeth, please.* While sometimes a light grazing with your chompers can actually feel quite pleasurable to him, more often than not, things will go awry (you know exactly what this means) and you may accidentally bite him. And there's no fun in that.
- *Don't forget your tongue.* Lots of tongue action is key, especially around the ridge at the tip and on the underside of the penis, which is ultrasensitive.
- *Keep it slick.* Don't be shy about saliva dripping out of your mouth and all over the place. The more the better.
- *Handle him well.* Grip one hand firmly around the base of his penis and move it up and down, in time with the motion of your mouth.
- *Twist your hand around.* But don't just go up and down, up and down. Move your hand in all directions—kind of like an "Indian burn" without the burn.
- *Be ambitious.* Cover the whole penis with your mouth, and the deeper you can take it in, the better.

The sensation of his penis hitting the back of your throat excites him.

- *Swallow.* If you can. There's nothing a man loves more. If you don't want to swallow, have him spray all over your tummy or breasts, or even your face if you are feeling particularly kinky. He will never stop thanking you for this. Just keep in mind: Gagging, choking, spitting it out, and running right to the bathroom afterward to wash it off can be big turn-offs for men. (If you find the idea of swallowing totally repugnant and need to spit, just don't make a big deal about it. Hold it in your mouth and discreetly spit into a towel kept at your bedside. If you want to try and improve the taste, see the "sweetening" Recipe for Success on page 75. It might just make the idea more, well, palatable.)

Frosty the Snow Woman

Here's a perfect game for a sweltering summer day. Have a glass of ice ready at your bedside, and also make an ice pack wrapped in a thin towel.

Take an ice cube into your mouth and go down on him, swirling the ice up and down his shaft with your tongue. Get him revved up and excited, but don't finish him. Not yet, at least. Instead, as you sense him getting close, stop and take a break. Take the ice pack and place it over your privates, and while you do, why not take another ice cube and roll it all over you—your nipples, your tummy, whatever feels good. Now take another ice cube into your mouth and make out passionately with your guy. When that ice melts, have him

Recipe for Success

If you don't like the taste of ejaculate, you're not alone. But if there was a recipe that would make it taste better, would you give it a try? About an hour before love-making, blend the following together:

2 tablespoons agave nectar
1 cup soy milk
1/4 teaspoon ground cinnamon
1/4 teaspoon ground ginger
1/4 teaspoon nutmeg
1/4 teaspoon ground cloves

Have him drink it down and see if you like the change. If you do, be sure to share the recipe with friends.

enter you and savor the crazy sensation of entering your frozen female parts.

The SBJ

This is short for spontaneous blow job. And what could be better or more kinky than to just surprise your honey out of the blue with a blow job? Something you give him for no other reason than that you love him, love his penis, and just want to make him feel good? Try this out while watching TV, in the middle of dinner—any time when he least expects it.

Cover your teeth with your lips and make sure they're moistened with a smooth gloss so you can easily slide those sexy lips of yours up and down his hot rod. Nibble on the sensitive ridge on the underside of his penis, flutter your tongue over the head, and then, as if on a Popsicle, continue lapping and licking, sucking and fluttering. Pucker your lips together and shake your head from right to left while pressing your lips against the head of his penis. He'll never know what hit him.

Under Cover Lover

Set your alarm clock for fifteen minutes earlier than usual and try not to disturb your partner. Well, at least not right away. . . . Slide yourself all the way under the covers and slink over to your man's manhood. Now gently take hold of it, stroking, caressing, licking, and kissing. Hold his penis so that it rests on the inside of your hand but your hands are open, lick your lips and push them up and down the shaft lengthwise, occasionally slipping his manhood inside your mouth, and then go back to tongue stroking. It will put a spring in his step for the rest of the day.

Pearl Necklace

A "pearl necklace" is when a man ejaculates around his lover's neck. Men are ultravisual and like to see the, well, fruits of their labor. So why not indulge him? You can either pleasure him to the point of ejaculation and make your own necklace, or have him masturbate over you. If you really want to be blatant about it, there's a ZZ Top song called "Pearl Necklace" you might consider playing in the background.

A LITTLE OF THIS, A LITTLE OF THAT

And finally . . . here are a few techniques for you both to enjoy.

Mirror, Mirror

Wherever the largest mirror in your house is, place a soft blanket down in front of it. Now both of you strip down—or

Seventy-one

Everyone knows what a 69 is—the act of simultaneously orally pleasing each other. So what makes up the other 2? A 71 incorporates 2 fingers while you're in a 69. Women: While you're orally pleasuring your partner in a 69, take your index finger and middle finger and massage his perineum—the little "bridge" between his anus and testicles. Massage the area and pulsate on it with your fingers—and even your tongue if you're feeling especially kinky. You might even penetrate his anus with your finger (or tongue), but that's entirely up to you and your comfort level. And for the men: One finger penetrates her vagina and the other either stimulates or penetrates her anus. Just be sure you use plenty of lube for anything penetrating such a sensitive area. Both women and men get an extra charge by having their anuses stimulated—and it doesn't mean your man is secretly gay. There are many sensitive nerve endings surrounding the anus, which enhance pleasure. If you're concerned about hygiene, don't perform this act until you've taken a shower, and even try using a condom over your finger and tongue. In the kinky realm, this one shoots way over to "wild," so if it's outside your comfort zone, don't worry. It doesn't mean you aren't kinky in other ways.

better yet, strip each other down. Be sure to have a bottle of your favorite lube handy. Now both of you sit in front of the mirror with your legs spread apart. Apply an ample amount of lube onto your genitals and begin self-pleasuring, keeping eye contact with your partner's reflection. Now, who will orgasm first? We've already talked about what a turn-on it is to watch your partner masturbate—and this takes it to a whole new level. The point of this game is that there are so many ways to share sexual experiences with each other—and you don't even have to be touching.

NOW YOU KNOW . . .

As you did before, that men and women derive pleasure from different techniques—but both can benefit from a good dose of kink. In the next chapter, we'll go over more of the basics as you add some kink to your sex positions. And then we'll enter the realm of pure fun and fearless kink.

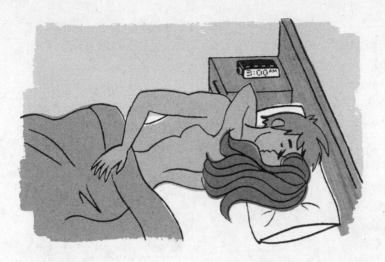

Chapter 5

I Put My Legs Where?

When's the last time you thought about sex positions? I mean, really thought about them? And even better, tried out something new and exotic and adventurous. That's what I thought. But don't worry—you're not alone. Any couple who's been together for a while is guilty of falling into a missionary-sex rut. And for good reason. Missionary is straightforward, simple, and doesn't necessarily require much agility or imagination. But is it kinky?

In this chapter, we'll go beyond the basics and then learn all kinds of exciting alternatives to the usual options (don't worry, these moves won't necessarily require advanced yoga training). As you engage in these fun, fantasy-fulfilling, and even fit-making sex-ercises, you'll find lots of playful alternatives to the basics. And you'll have a really great time together while you're at it.

The positions here are intended only as a guide. You'll be surprised how you can kink up any sex position with just a little imagination. Can missionary sex be kinky? You bet. All it takes is a little creativity, a healthy dose of connection, and a whole lotta love. There's nothing more satisfying in sex than fully connecting with your partner. And kinky can do just that. Even if it means being twisted into a pretzel.

> ### Naughty Nibble
>
> You can always make time for sex—including the middle of the night. Instead of worrying about work deadlines or mounting bills as you lie awake in bed at three in the morning, why not go for a quickie? You'll be back to blissful sleep in no time.

TIME AFTER TIME

They say the average sex session lasts fifteen to twenty minutes. But surely you have more time than that for your partner. In this exercise, you'll see just how long you can last. Tonight, place a timer at your bedside, preferably in a spot where you can reach it without getting up. Set the timer for fifteen minutes and don't do anything at all—at least not at first. Lie together naked and don't touch. Instead, start to fantasize about what you want to do with each other. You can do this silently while making intense eye contact, or you can even talk it through.

When the timer runs out, set it for another fifteen minutes. This time, you can start touching. You can kiss, you can stroke, you can hold each other close. He can stimulate her clitoris with the tip of his penis, which can be teasingly satisfying for both partners. But absolutely no penetration is permitted. Now set the timer for another fifteen minutes. It's okay to go almost all the way. He may enter her, but with no thrusting or grinding of any kind. Instead, kiss, cuddle, stroke, and enjoy being close while you are connected in such an intimate way. And when the timer goes off again, you now have my blessing to go totally wild. But can you last another fifteen minutes before you just have to orgasm?

LEGS STAY TOGETHER

Here's another way to make missionary a bit more interesting. She lies on her back, and instead of opening her legs to accept him, she keeps them closed, meaning he's going to have to squeeze himself in. The result? Excellent friction for all. This is a great position for clitoral stimulation. To make the best of it, before he enters, he should rub the tip of his penis against her clitoris—back and forth, around and around, side to side. During lovemaking, he pulls out at random and continues to stimulate her with the tip. Add a dab of Nympho's Desire (see Resources for suppliers) on her clit to take it up a notch. She continues to keep her legs closed as tightly as she can manage as he thrusts inside of her. This is also a great technique for rear-entry positions—but we'll get into that in a bit.

TO A T

Part of the thrill of missionary for a woman is the absolute sense of being "taken." So why not make the most of the sumptuous sensation of submission? Here, both partners are in their standard missionary poses. Her legs can be up or down—it doesn't matter. It's her arms we're dealing with here. Once inside her, he grabs her hands and stretches her arms out so her body essentially forms a T shape. With her arms pinned down, she is unable to control anything that happens to her—she cannot push him away or pull him closer. Her pleasure, in essence, is all in his hands. To make the position even more intimate, he should kiss her neck and across her "wingspan," from one side to the other.

WHO'S IN CHARGE?

Here's a tricky and fun position that's excellent for stimulating the G-spot. In it, she lies flat on her back, bends her knees, and holds them together. She raises her butt slightly and he kneels under it, so that her butt rests on the fronts of his thighs. She opens her legs at the knees and places one foot over each of his shoulders. She can support herself either by keeping her hands on the bed or by placing pillows under her back. His hands remain free and can hold her waist, which is a very sexy, manly, take-charge way to control the thrusting.

THE SCISSOR

Sure, spooning is fun, but what about the rest of the utensil drawer? When it comes to over-the-edge sexy positioning, with maximum penetration and stimulation, nothing beats the scissor. In this kinky variation of the classic position, she lies with her tush at the edge of the bed, her legs straight up in the air. If the bed is low, a pillow may be placed underneath her butt to give her some "height." He enters her and begins thrusting lightly. As he thrusts, he holds her ankles in his hands and begins scissoring her legs by crossing them and opening them, crossing and opening.

Most women love it when a man takes control, and this is a hugely controlling position for him. The movement of her

Just for Him . . .

Many men move from initial penetration to mad thrusting instantly, but why? Did you know that most women actually find the first sensation of penetration to be one of the most exciting aspects of sex? In fact, it feels really good for both parties, so why stop at once when you can enjoy the sensation over and over again? The next time you enter your lover, thrust only once. Then stop, pull out, and give some attention to her other sensitive parts, like her breasts and nipples. Then enter her again; then pull out. Move downtown and work your magic touch. Then stop and penetrate her again; and then pull out. Do this as many times as both of you can withstand, and you will both come quickly and powerfully.

legs, controlled by him, stimulates the vaginal walls as well as the entrance to the vagina, and also creates varied pressure on the penis. It's also a deep, penetrating, high-friction position—which no man would ever object to. Repeat as needed—until she explodes in ecstasy.

THE CUL-DE-SAC O

Did you know that women can have cervical orgasms? Now you guys do. At the bottom of the cervix there's an area sexologists call the "cul-de-sac," essentially a bundle of nerves that when properly stimulated actually produces cul-de-sac orgasms. Here's a great way to get or give one. First find a relatively low surface for her to lie on, as this only works if she is lying lower than his hips: He stands on the floor facing her; she lies on her back, with her tush at the edge of the bed or couch or wherever you've ended up. When done correctly, she will experience plenty of pleasure; but if he thrusts too hard against the cervix, it could possibly cause her pain or discomfort—and there's no fun in that. Remember that this is a deep-penetration position, so when he enters, he should do so gently, aiming his penis downward. On the first stroke, just before pulling back, he grinds his hips around in circles repeatedly, kind of in a stirring motion. And oh the pleasure he will be stirring up for you both.

THE SWITCHBACK

The what? Don't worry—it's not as complicated as it seems. In this position, she lies on her back with her legs together. He approaches and enters her slowly for ten long thrusts (long meaning counting to three going in and counting to three pulling out). Next, switch back to standard missionary, in which her legs are wrapped around him, and take ten shorter thrusts. Now switch back (get it now?): Her legs are together, the thrusts are longer, and then, yes, switch back. . . . Repeat this back-and-forth several times until she explodes into orgasm.

JUST OFF CENTER

Self-pleasuring is mandatory for her before trying out this position. Why? Because this position is especially for couples who know which side of her clitoris is the most sensitive. That's right, ladies. For some women, one side of the clitoris has more nerve endings and thus is more sensitive. So it's time for some, well, independent study—if both don't already know which side it is.

In this position, she lies on her back and bends her legs,

keeping them together. She lifts them over either his left or right shoulder, the opposite shoulder of the side of her clitoris that is most sensitive, and keeps her knees and thighs pressed together as he thrusts. For example, if the left side of her clitoris is more sensitive, she'll put her legs over his right shoulder, and vice versa. Because she is getting more friction on one side or the other, she will get the stimulation she needs to climax that much faster.

LEFT, RIGHT, LEFT

This maneuver can be done in many positions, but it seems to work best in missionary. Probably because that's when he has the most balance and control. Once inside her, he aims his penis first to the left side of the vagina for three long strokes, and then takes three more strokes to the right. Then three to the left, then three to the right, and so on. When not in missionary, she can take the reins, changing the angle of her pelvis as he enters her—even while lying in the typically submissive position of being on her back. The rhythm it creates is guaranteed to rock both partners' worlds.

RIDING SHOTGUN

Drive around and find a secluded spot, with her behind the wheel (this one's all about her being in control). When the car is safely in park (we're looking for a dangerous thrill here—not a stupid-dangerous one) and the ignition turned

Naughty Nibble

Just because one side of her clitoris may be more sensitive than the other doesn't mean that's the side both partners need to focus on all the time. A little teasing by stimulating the other side—and coming oh so close to grazing the sensitive part—will go a long way in prolonging ecstasy.

Just for Her . . .

Get out a pair of old jeans, preferably ones he hates because they're too baggy and saggy and should be destroyed anyway. Now, with a scissor, cut a slit at the crotch. Now slip them on over your naked tush—that's right, no undies. Tie a sweatshirt around your waist so he doesn't notice and try to act normal. Now do something totally average, like sit on the couch together and watch TV. While you're watching, lean over and tell him you'd like to sit on his lap. Or, even better, just do it. Innocently lift yourself onto his lap, facing him (though if you're very coordinated, you could sit facing away from him). Then, not so innocently, unzip his pants, pull out his member, and tell him you've always wanted to do it with your jeans on. Slide his penis right through the slit you've cut and rock back and forth, balancing yourself by holding the back of the chair or couch.

---

off, she climbs over, straddles him, and rides him into the sunset. Not only will endorphins be high with the thrill of possibly getting caught, it's a highly orgasmic position for her. Tip: She should plan ahead for this one and wear a dress or skirt—anything that can be quickly pushed aside.

THE ZOMBIE

Can zombies be sexy? In this sex position, damn straight they can. In it, one of the partners lies there, lifeless, while the other goes crazy all over his or her body—and brings his or her partner back to life. This is a "take-charge" situation right from the get-go, so if you've ever considered dabbling in domination, it's a great place to start.

Dominating partner: Tell your lover to lie back and let him know that he is absolutely forbidden to move for the duration. Remove his clothing, piece by piece. Tease. Flirt. Caress. Stroke. Kiss. Lick. Now remove your clothes, piece by piece. Use a little massage oil to slick you both up and slide your naked body all over his. Take extra time to arouse those parts that are most sensitive. Pretend that you will soon end this amorous agony by making her think you'll be entering. Then don't. If they try to move, to touch you, to angle in a new position, remind your partner that this is forbidden. Kiss, suck, and lick every place you've always wanted to. Then bring your partner to orgasm with your hands or mouth, or through intercourse. Still, they are not permitted to touch you or move in any way. All your partner is allowed to do is come. It's a delightful dose of domination sure to delight even the shyest submissive. (And if you like this, there's lots more fun to be had in Chapter 8.)

> ## Naughty Nibble
>
> Most women have their best orgasms while on top because they can move around and control the entry, the angle of the penis, and the speed of the thrusts. This way, the G-spot can be hit every time.

MILK AND WATER EMBRACE

Think of the Kama Sutra as ancient kink—but just as fun to experiment with today as it was thousands of years ago. The Milk and Water Embrace is just one of the super-kinky positions that come from the granddaddy of all sex manuals that you'll find in this chapter. And it's also one of my personal favorites. In this woman-on-top position, he sits on the edge of the bed with his legs hanging over the side, his back on the mattress, and his feet on the floor. But it's okay if his feet don't quite reach. She straddles him, facing him, her hands planted on the bed by his shoulders, her knees on each side of his pelvis, her feet alongside his legs—and perhaps adorned in a pair of spiky heels. She can also kneel over him on the bed, or, if she's especially strong and, um, springy, she can squat over him. Whatever you choose, it's an exciting way for her to take charge and give him the ride of his life.

BUTTER CHURN

Why on earth would a butter churn be considered sexy? In this position, it's all about the motion. It goes like this: He sits, legs apart, on the edge of the bed or in a chair or even on the floor—whatever's comfortable and provides the best balance. She gets on top of him, facing him, her legs wrapped tightly around him. He places his hands on her waist, and instead of the usual "in and out motion," she instead rotates and grinds on top of him, like a butter churn, as he helps maneuver her. And you don't even have to be Amish to enjoy it.

> ### Naughty Nibble
> Keep kissing during sex (if the position you're in allows, of course), and get ready for more intense orgasms, as this lets you maintain a powerful emotional connection while you ride, thrust, and grind.

THE BIG SQUEEZE

In this intimate sex position, the best place for him to sit is on a stool. She sits on top of him, facing him, with her legs wrapped around his waist. He places one hand on her back and the other on her tush. Before you begin grinding away, she simply squeezes his pubis muscles by Kegeling—at least twenty times—as both partners enjoy the sensation. When it becomes too much to stand, by all means start having sex. Just keep squeezing while you do.

(SL)EASY CHAIR

The majority of women like high-intimacy sexual positions, and this is definitely one of those. You could do this on the bed, but it works much better on a big, roomy chair. He sits in the chair and she slips onto his lap, facing him, and straddles him. Now she leans back and puts her legs over his shoulders, letting them drape over the back of the chair. He holds on tight to her hips as both partners get a workout, rocking back and forth. When he aims his penis toward her navel, mind-blowing G-spot stimulation will be the delicious result.

RIDE 'EM HIGH

In the realm of woman-on-top positions, The Cowgirl is queen. In it, he lies down on the bed or on the floor and she mounts him. But instead of kneeling, she squats. Then, just when you thought it couldn't get more she-dominated, she turns around, facing away from his head, and she rides like a wild woman right into the sunset. Stay in character, with the yee-hahs and all. Add a cowboy hat, chaps, and some cowboy boots and you'll be ready for the bedroom rodeo.

Just for Him . . .

The next time you're making hot passionate love to your partner (which should be tonight, by the way), give her a good tease. Just as she begins to climax, and before you come, quickly take out your penis. She may be annoyed, confused, or shocked, but what she doesn't realize is that you're doing her a huge favor. As quickly and suddenly as you slipped out, push yourself back in and keep thrusting till completion. For many women, the interruption builds the sexual tension and will actually add to the strength of the orgasm.

THE GOAT'S POSTURE

In this position, also from the Kama Sutra, she lies on her side and stretches out her bottom leg. He crouches himself down between her thighs, kneels inside the bottom leg, and lifts her top leg over his back. Now he enters and thrusts, all the while supporting her arms and shoulders.

SIDE-STEPPIN'

In this side-entry variation, she lies on her back with a small pillow placed under her butt. Her legs are raised. He lies on his side, perpendicular to her. One leg is straight, one leg bent, and the bent leg hovers over one of her legs, creating an X. She can keep her legs up in the air, and as she becomes tired, she can relax her legs and bring them down.

THE HIP-HUGGER

Another one of my personal favorite positions, the Hip-Hugger is like Side-Steppin'—with a twist. In it he lies on his side, she on her back, perpendicular to him, her legs bent at the knees over his pelvis. She then swings both legs over his hips, giving his penis direct access. As neither partner is worried about balancing, each can use their two free hands to stimulate each other, massaging whatever feels good.

THE TUSH PUSH

The next time you make love in the doggie-style position (rear-entry vaginal, not anal), try this exciting maneuver. As he thrusts inside, he reaches around to her front and stimulates her clitoris as he kisses up and down her neck. As one hand continues stimulating her clitoris, he, with his free hand, lightly grabs her butt cheek and pushes it out to the side. Now, with every thrust he makes, he pushes her tush to the side. As we'll get into in later chapters, many people enjoy a little butt stimulation, and this is a pretty good, conservative way to try it out and see how it feels. It truly makes for some interesting sensations.

BARK AND PURR

Most people enjoy sex doggie style on some level, but as stimulating and satisfying as rear-entry vaginal sex can be for him, it can sometimes be uncomfortable for her. Some women derive no pleasure from it at all, mostly because the way he enters her is more uncomfortable or even painful than anything else. Here are two ways to vary the classic doggie-style position that can make it more pleasurable for her. In the first variation, she keeps her legs together, with his on the outside. In the second, she keeps her legs apart but rests her arms, head, and chest on a pillow, with her tush up in the air. To really enhance the experience, he should not just pound away at her. He should gently stroke her shoulders and breasts, kiss her neck and face when she turns around, her mouth.

THE SLAMMY SLIDE

Warning: This one's only for the most limber and physically fit and is especially not recommended if either partner has back problems. I named this for one of my wild friends, who just loves it. In it, he stands upright while she stands with her back toward him. Now she bends slightly at the knees and then over at the waist, until her bottom is facing up. He then places both his hands on her butt cheeks to balance her and enters her. He has to support her or she may end up rolling over—which will probably make you both crack up. Which wouldn't be so bad really. Because what's great sex without a few good laughs, anyway?

THE DOGHOUSE

Usually, being "in the doghouse" is not where you want to be. But here, it's the best. Decide you're going to make love tonight in the doggie-style position but not climax—neither of you. When either of you gets close to orgasm, stop and breathe deeply, keeping his penis inside. Resume sex, thrusting slowly. There's no rush and there's no goal. The next time either one of you gets close to orgasm, stop again. With his penis still inside, hold each other and just relax, enjoying the comfort and the closeness. After a while, resume what you were doing, but, again, don't come. It takes a lot of discipline not to come, but it's well worth the closeness you're creating and the sensations you're going to experience when you finally do release.

SUSPENDED CONGRESS

Not a political thing but another delightful position from the Kama Sutra, this is a chal-

> ### naughty nibble
>
> When you wake up tomorrow morning, tell your partner you don't have a headache. For the rest of the day, remind them of the same thing and be playful about it. When it comes time for bed, strip down, snuggle up, and remind them again. If they don't catch on, take matters into your own hands and show them just what not having a headache means.

lenging standing position that should be attempted only by the most physically fit. In it, he stands against a wall for support. She faces him, wrapping her arms around his neck. Now she jumps up, wrapping her thighs around his waist, with her knees bent and feet resting on the wall up at his waist level. She controls the action, rocking back and forth and pushing her feet against the wall.

THE BREAST SEX YOU EVER HAD

This is an especially erotic turn-on for "breast men." In it, she lies on her back and he pours massage oil all over her breasts. Both rub it in. He also lubes up his penis. Now he straddles her, placing his penis between her breasts as she holds them together, sandwiching his member. Size doesn't matter here; all that matters is the sensation generated as he slides his penis back and forth between her breasts. It's up to both parties where he finishes—her breasts, her tummy, even her face if both parties are feeling especially kinky.

NOW YOU KNOW . . .

Even the most standard position can sizzle when you infuse it with a little kink. Now that we've covered the basics and seen all kinds of ways to spice them up, it's time to cross over into the realm of "Kinkier and Kinkier" and see how far you're willing to go.

> ### Naughty Nibble
> The "refractory period" is the time between when a man first ejaculates and is ready to go again. On average, it's about thirty minutes, but varies due to age, level of fitness, and other factors. To shorten the refractory period, leave his penis inside after he ejaculates and wait for it to become erect again—usually this is less than a few minutes.

Kinkier and Kinkier

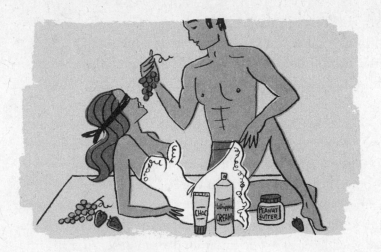

Chapter 6

Tasty, Tantalizing Fun with Food

Some of the best sex happens when it's just you and your partner, exploring, savoring, devouring each other. But sex can also be fantastic when you add a little texture and flavor into the mix—literally. Not comfy with the idea of food in the bed? Maybe it's not for everyone, but don't let that sway you from trying out some of the fun tips in this chapter. You can lay down an old comforter over your bedding, or even place a plastic sheet under that if you think it's necessary. But, if possible, just let go. Seriously. Take a deep breath and banish all of your worries and inhibitions from your bedroom. Yes, food can be messy and hard to control. But isn't the best sex you've ever had just that? So try to let go of your hang-ups and just enjoy.

In this chapter, we'll transform your boring old grocery shopping routine into something sexy. We'll look at traditional aphrodisiacs, foods that are just plain sexy, and ones you probably already have on hand just waiting to be put to good use.

More than any oyster or square of chocolate or strawberry, always keep in mind that enthusiasm is the ultimate aphrodisiac. And, as we're learning, there are so many ways to show enthusiasm, subtle and overt. The enthusiasm and openness you share as you endeavor to frolic with food—or other kinky options coming later in this book—will not only raise your level of eroticism around the house, they'll help you build erotic memories that get you through the hard times . . . if you ever have any after this book.

9½ WEEKS—AND COUNTING

Everyone remembers the classic scene in *9½ Weeks* during which Mickey Rourke playfully tortures and tantalizes Kim Basinger with treats from the fridge. This movie is a staple of kinkiness, with so many scenes to reenact and enjoy (toned down to a level you're comfortable with, of course). We'll get into this movie and others a bit more later, but in a chapter about sex and food, this scene cannot be overlooked.

One of the elements of this scene that made it so sexy is the blindfold. The element of surprise really made for an explosive, obsession-sparking sexual experience for Kim Basinger's character. She never knew what he would be touching her with next.

For that reason, when you act out this scene in front of your own fridge (and long after your kids have gone to bed,

Grocery Run

The following foods have been said to stir the libido, so be sure to include some of them on the dinner menu tonight—and keep your favorites always in abundance in your kitchen:

- Lobster
- Raw oysters
- Sushi
- Caviar
- Artichokes

- Avocados
- Bananas
- Cucumbers
- Watermelon
- Almonds

- Chocolate
- Ginger
- Olive oil
- Honey
- Wine

or, even better, on a night they're out), don't forget the blind-fold. A bandanna, a silk scarf, anything you have lying around will do. It doesn't have to completely obscure your lover's vision—just enough so that they don't know what surprise is coming next.

Lay down a blanket or comforter in front of the fridge—but not something that needs to be dry-cleaned, because the fun of this game is that it gets m-e-s-s-y. Make sure your refrigerator is packed with finger foods, like strawberries, grapes, and cubes of cheese, and don't forget the foods that are fun to lick away, like chocolate syrup and whipped cream. . . .

Guide your lover to your erotic picnic. Start out on the tame side, perhaps feeding him a simple grape or dipping a strawberry into the chocolate syrup and gently placing it in her mouth. Take some whipped cream into your own mouth and give your lover a passionate kiss, or dab a little on your lover's nipples or tummy. Gently lick it away with the tip of

Fun with Fetishes: Food

Fetishes run the gamut from tame to wild, but really they are simple. Sometimes something that isn't necessarily sexual makes you feel that way. Here are some common food-related fetishes I've encountered in my practice.

Milk Fetish

I once worked with a couple who were into playing with milk. The man liked watching his partner drink it, then spew it from her mouth all over her breasts. Sometimes they would even take milk baths together. If that sounds like something that might turn you on, have a few gallons of milk at the ready by the bathtub and get ready to play!

Chocolate Fetish

Chocolate is a common fetish—and we surely use a lot of chocolate in this chapter. There's now a product available on the market called Smooches, which is a delicious body dust that comes in all kinds of flavors, including chocolate. You can use this magic dust on your partner, sprinkling it wherever you please and licking it away. You can "paint" your lover with melted chocolate or chocolate syrup. You can think of inventive ways to use chocolate "statues"—maybe giving the concept of "the Rabbit" (see page 127) a whole new meaning with a solid chocolate bunny.

Cheese Fetish

There really is something for everyone. I actually have a guy friend who loves grated cheese so much, he likes to sprinkle it all over his girlfriend and eat it off whichever part of her it's dropped on. Proof that sometimes "cheesy" can be totally sexy.

Sticky Fetish

The sensation of "sticky" is one that turns quite a few people on—and food provides the best opportunity to experience it. A word of warning: This is *super messy,* but if you really like this kind of thing, just be prepared: Lay down a plastic tarp. Two super-sticky foods are honey and peanut butter—and they actually taste really good mixed together. Squirt one another with the honey. Slather on the peanut butter with your hands. Once you're covered, you can rub up against each other and test the stickiness. And when you're done with that, enjoy licking it off each other

your tongue. Be inventive about where you dab the whipped cream or pour the chocolate syrup, taking your time before you get to the "main course." When neither of you can stand it any longer, go ahead and go to town. All the time you took leading up to the big event may mean your lover will be right on the brink—so now bring him or her over the edge. And what could be more delicious than that?

MENTHOL MANIA

You don't need to be sick to benefit from the tingly sensations menthol provides. Place a couple of mentholated cough drops in your mouth, swirl them around, then spit them out. Now make out with your partner, asking your sweetie if he or she is enjoying the sensation of menthol in their mouth—and tell them that you'd like to try to see where else this tingly-ness might feel especially good. Now swirl a couple more in your mouth and this time leave them in. Head south on your partner, tickling, teasing, and tingling as you lap, lick, and suck away.

CURIOUSLY POTENT

Here's a trick sure to impress and delight. Swirl a couple of Altoids in your mouth before going down on your partner. Leave them in your mouth and give him a thrill, with both the tingles from the Altoids as well as the added sensation of the actual mints. Now take it up a notch. Remove your warm, wet mouth and make it a real blow job as you lightly blow on the area you just licked. Now bring back that warm, tingly mouth of yours. Now come up for air and blow again. Repeat this exercise at least ten times for a curiously intense experience for you both.

WATERMELON DREAMS

Nothing cools you down when you're hot like a nice serving of ice-cold watermelon, so why not whip it out when you're feeling hot . . . and bothered? Trace your lover's body parts with watermelon chunks and lick the luscious sweet trails you make. Run the watermelon over chest and tummy, lips and cheeks, nipples and privates. Yum, yum.

STRAWBERRY FIELDS FOREVER

There are not many foods sexier than strawberries. They're sweet and succulent—not to

Naughty Nibble

The orgasm should not be the be-all and end-all of your sexual experience. To make it such puts too much pressure on the woman to climax, which actually impedes her ability to do so. Enjoy pleasure for pleasure's sake, whether you prolong the ecstasy with massage or, in this case, foodplay. The orgasm is just the icing on the cake.

mention fun to eat and feed. Here's a new way to have some fun with them, inspired by the famous Beatles song.

Take a handful of strawberries and slice them very thin. Have your partner lie naked on their back and "plant" them all over their body as your partner relaxes, enjoying the sensation of wet and cold provided by the strawberries—and full of delicious anticipation for what comes next.

Strategically arrange the slices in the shape of a heart, a circle, an X. Whatever inspires you. Now eat them up. Start with the strawberries you planted in the most innocent places and tease all the way to the hottest spots. By the time you get there, your partner will be absolutely ravenous and desperate to devour you.

PEACHES AND CREAM

I've taught more classes in giving fabulous oral sex than anything else, and I'm always amazed how couples don't properly communicate what they truly want. I decided to make it fun and easy by bringing in select fruits, which you can easily do at home, too.

To teach him, I cut a peach in half and hand her the half with the pit. I tell them to think of the pit as the clit and the fruit around it as the labia. You get it. Next I tell her to lick and suck the peach the way she would like her partner to lick and suck her. It probably

Just for Her . . .

Tonight, teach your partner the true meaning of the term "peppermint stick." Suck on a peppermint and, keeping it in your mouth, go down on him. With your tongue, roll it up and down his shaft, sucking and swirling the peppermint as you move up and down with your mouth. Try to flick it around his penis as you keep the peppermint in your mouth—just be careful not to choke. Then hold the peppermint in your front teeth and rub the tip of the mint back and forth around the ridge of his penis. He'll never think of candy canes in quite the same way again.

comes as no surprise to learn that many men find this sex-ercise more than a little arousing. Then, on his half, he re-peats what he's been taught as she guides him one way or the other. And then it's her turn.

Next comes the most obvious food prop: a banana. Now he's supposed to show her what he wants, and then she's supposed to repeat it on her fruit. However, you'd be sur-prised how many straight guys will not do this. Instead, she does it, and he guides her as she goes. He might not actually demonstrate for himself, but most men are comfortable telling women what they want as the women demonstrate on the banana. Of course, in the privacy of your own bedroom, who knows what he'll be willing to do.

> ## Just for Her . . .
>
> Drink two glasses of pineapple juice at least two hours before getting hot and heavy with your partner. Many women swear this makes them taste delicious down there.

THE JUICER

Shake up your morning routine by ditching your juicer. It's time to try out a juicer you never knew you had. Okay, admittedly, this will not be for everyone. But for those ad-venturous enough to give it a shot . . . well, let's just say you'll never look at citrus in the same way ever again.

Cut a hole in an orange from one end to the other, wide enough to accommodate his penis. You may want to put a condom on for this, as oranges are acidic and the juice could burn his sensitive shaft. Now slip his shaft—erect or not, it doesn't matter—through the hole. Manipulate the orange up and down over his penis, circling it as if using a juicer. Now alternate the pressure you squeeze him with—one hard squeeze followed by a bunch of little pulsating squeezes. As the juice pours, lick up every drop—no matter where it goes.

CHERRY TOMATO

You can have a lot of fun with something as innocent as a bowl of cherry tomatoes. I recommend this kind of tomato because the size is just right for you to control and the round shape is much easier to roll than the oval shape of a grape tomato. (You could also use frozen grapes for this technique.)

Blindfold (yes, the blindfold again) your partner and make sure he or she's nice and comfy, lying faceup. Now take one of those tomatoes—straight from the fridge, please, as cold is better here—and with the palm of your hand roll it over her arms, nipples, up and down her legs, her ankles, her forehead . . .

Now have him or her flip over and turn your attention to his shoulders, back, the backs of his legs, his gorgeous tush. Roll a cold tomato up and down her labia, and around her clit. Take two tomatoes in hand and palm his penis with that hand. As the tomatoes warm, reach for new ones. It's going to make your partner crazy as he or she tries to figure out what you're pleasuring them with . . . but never tell. If she guesses, treat her to a sexual favor of her choosing. Just don't give in until she does. And if she continues to guess wrong, then she owes you a favor for each missed guess.

HOT DIGGETY DOG

Okay, this one's maybe even a bit beyond kinky, but it's also absolutely hilarious. It may seem a little strange, but I promise you that couples I've coached who've tried this rave about it as being one of their favorites—and probably because it's so bizarre.

What's for dinner, honey? Tonight is Hot Dog Night. Put out all your favorite condiments and cook up some hot dogs. Have a couple, but be sure to save a bun or two—and do not toast it. Guys, you can try asking your woman to do this, but this may be one of those things she'll feel more comfortable suggesting. So, girls, get to it.

Suggest to your man that you'd like to sample his weiner and tell him to whip it out. Slip it in a bun and dress it in your favorite condiments. Now lick up the ketchup or mustard or mayo and nibble the bun. You can actually even use the bun as a kind of sex toy, squeezing it up and down his "hot dog," licking the tip every time it pops up over the top of the bun. Be as creative as you want—and remember that this is *supposed* to be ridiculous. Just have fun with it.

A BEDROOM BANQUET

Tonight why not whip together a meal that can be served and savored using only your fingers. . . . That doesn't necessarily mean you have to limit the menu to traditional finger foods. Think texture here. What foods give you the most pleasure when you experience them? If it gets messy, so what. It only means licking it up where it falls—and hopefully that will be someplace really good.

And the fun doesn't have to wait till dinnertime. Whip up a sexy menu and leave it in your lover's briefcase or pocketbook. It could read like this:

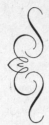
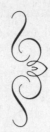

BEDROOM BANQUET

Our bedroom, tonight.
Please join me for a decadent dinner in bed,
guaranteed to delight all your senses. Come
hungry. Clothing optional. . . .

As you prepare the room, amp up the romance. Light candles. Drape the bed with soft linens—preferably ones that are machine washable. Line up all the foods on a tray—and don't forget dessert. Perhaps some chocolate-covered strawberries or truffles? A decadent crème brûlée? Just remember, whatever you serve, leave the utensils in the kitchen and enjoy the sensation of licking food—and having food licked—from your fingertips. And who knows how inventive you can be with body parts and food service.

MILK SHAKE

This shake trick takes the cake . . . and the ice-cream topping. Tell your lover you feel like going out for milk shakes tonight—but that you really want to enjoy them at home. In bed. Your lover will probably not suspect that this is a seduction trick. What's more innocent than a milk shake?

When you get your treats, bring it to the next level, telling your lover that your milk shake will taste better for you if he or she is naked and lying down. They may look at you like you're crazy, but convince them to go with it.

Take your straw in your mouth and suck up just enough creamy goodness to fill the straw. Now, using your tongue to manipulate the liquid, stand over your lover's body, pointing the end of the straw strategically. Release small drops of the liquid on your lover's body—one at a time, please. Drop a bit on a nipple and lick it off. Aim for the belly button and lap it up. Think of all your lover's hot spots and "cool" them down. Just be sure that wherever you drop those droplets, you're licking off the ice cream and leaving a sweet warm kiss in its place.

Swirl some milk shake in your mouth and kiss your lover deeply and sexily, giving him a taste of yours. When you're down to the last sip, use it to chill your mouth and go down on your partner, giving your lover a dessert he or she will never forget.

THE PAINT JOB

Speaking of hot spots . . . Here's an exercise that invites you and your partner to explore and discover ones you may not even have known you've had by "painting" them with chocolate. You'll need a small paintbrush, the size you'd use on a paint-by-numbers canvas. Though if you really like your chocolate, bring out the housepainter's brush and a nice-size bowl of chocolate syrup. Think cereal bowl. Hershey's chocolate syrup works well, and Kama Sutra Milk Chocolate body paint is even better (see Resources). If you'd like to make your own, here's my recipe: Pour 1¼ cups heavy cream in a bowl with 3 cups chocolate chips and melt in the microwave. Add a pinch of red pepper spice. Then stir, cool slightly, and apply. (Peppers increase circulation and stimulate nerve endings; chocolate contains two substances that are mood lifters.)

For women and men both, the alternating sensations of

the tickling from the brush, the gooey sensation of the chocolate, and, the best part, the warm, silky wetness of your mouth are guaranteed pleasure-triggers.

How to Paint a Naked Man

Dab the brush into the bowl of chocolate syrup and get it good and drenched. Take the brush and begin painting parts of his body you know are sensitive—his nipples, his shoulders, his neck. Paint a stroke and lick it off, or get him nice and covered and yummy first—whatever you both prefer.

Now that he's all worked up, head for his penis and "paint" it with long strokes, from base to tip. Be sure to really coat the shaft in all that luscious chocolate goodness. If it starts getting messy, no need to bother with a washcloth or wet paper towel; simply control and contain the mess by gently licking away stray drops as they fall. Not happy with your work or think you can do better? Then by all means, take a do-over. He won't complain. Lick the shaft squeaky clean and reapply the chocolate. Lick it clean again.

If both partners are willing, expand your working area to include the testicles and the "P-spot," aka the perineum, the area between his testicles and anus and a hugely sensitive part of him. Lick it off and reapply until he just can't take it anymore. Now take his whole member in your mouth and finish him off.

How to Paint a Naked Woman

With your brush carefully covered in chocolate, take long, luxurious strokes all over her body—and not just the obvious parts. Move out of the basic routine and test out her knees, her toes. Painting and licking her nipples will bring you both

Just for Him . . .

Here's a luscious, licking trick I learned from a lipstick lesbian. Have your partner lie down naked on the bed. Ask her to close her eyes, and when she does, strategically place flat-style lollipops on her naked body—one on each nipple, one on her tummy, one you know where . . . Now tease her everywhere as you lick around the lollipops. Here's the clincher: She isn't allowed to move. If she does, and in doing so knocks off one of the lollipops, the game reverses and she must do the same to you. And when the last lolly is licked, that's when the real fun begins.

enormous pleasure, but what about her wrists, palms, and fingertips?

Head south—but not *there* just yet. Take your chocolatey tool and brush her inner thighs, delicately lapping up the sexy syrup with the tip of your tongue. Now head for her labia. Delicately brush the syrup on both sides of her clit, but don't touch her there—not yet. . . . With gentle strokes, paint and lick, paint and lick, up and down, side to side. Now dab her clit and flick your tongue back and forth, just grazing the top. Add more chocolate and increase the intensity of your licks. Now forget the chocolate and give her what she's going to be desperate for just about now. Talk about decadent.

MARSHMALLOW MADNESS

Texture can command a huge and exciting role in sexplay—and not many things are as intriguing in texture as a marshmallow. Just be sure to get the regular-size ones and leave the minis for your hot chocolate. Smaller is definitely not better in this instance.

Strip down your partner and tell him to lie back and close his eyes. Start with his face, rolling one over his eyelids, cheeks, lips. Move down his body, rolling the marshmallow across his chin, over his ears, down his neck. Take another and roll it over his nipples, licking up the trail of marshmallow dust left behind. Roll another marshmallow down the length of his torso and around his belly button, then roll one just above the line where his pubic hair starts.

Now head for the finish line, taking another marshmallow and rolling it around the base of his manhood as if it were a third testicle. (And then roll it around those.) Or, for her, take the marshmallow and roll it up and down, side to side, over her clit. It will feel as good for her down there as the head of your penis—the textures are very close.

How coordinated are you? Put it to the test. Place a marshmallow in your mouth and take the head of his penis in your mouth. This is super-kinky, as it will almost feel like having two in your mouth at once. . . . Even if that kind of fantasy isn't for you, the sensation he will feel between your tongue and the marshmallow working him at once will make him explode in no time.

To please the ladies requires a touch more coordination for him—and can intensify her pleasure hugely. Guys: See if you can balance the marshmallow up against her clit with your upper lip. Keep it pressed there as you use your tongue to lick up and down her labia, using your fingers as well. It's like having three hands—or two tongues. . . . And just imagine how all that action will intensify and enhance her reaction.

HONEY DUST

What are all the truly kinky couples "buzzing" about? It's honey dust, a sweet golden powder guaranteed to sprinkle a

Naughty Nibble

Ever thought of Twizzlers as a sex toy? Tuck a couple lengthwise between her labia, one on each side. Then lick away at them, "missing" them almost every time as you treat her to some luscious licks. For him, hold a couple against his shaft and lick them up and down, making sure you use your tongue flat and wide so you're licking lots more than the licorice. Mmmm, mmm.

good dose of sensuality on your next lovemaking session. The best part is that it comes complete with a "duster" you can use to get the good stuff all over your lover's naked body. Dust all at once or just a bit at a time. Powder up her inner arms and the backs of her knees. Lightly dust her nipples, tummy, and between her legs. Dust his sexy broad shoulders. His pecs. The line that runs from his belly button to the base of his penis—and beyond. Now lick it off with soft, teasing laps. Not only will it feel absolutely wonderful for your lover, it also tastes great for you. Find this kinky powder at your local sex shop or order it online (see Resources).

CANDY TOSS

Before dinner tonight, place some M&Ms or Life Savers into a bowl next to your bed. After you eat, tell your partner you'd like to have dessert in the bedroom tonight, and that he or she should meet you there in five minutes.

When you get to the bedroom, strip off all your clothes and lie on the bed. Reach for the bowl and sprinkle the candy on those parts of your body you'd like their mouth to get closer to. Don't be too obvious about it. It's a delicious tease to give parts of you that don't always get erotic attention a little loving. Instead of going right for the grand prize, toss some of the candies around your belly button, on the area just above your pubes, maybe your wrists, the underside of your arm, the inside of your elbow—try to hit all your erogenous zones. Important: Insist that your partner also lick these areas clean so you won't be all sticky afterward. It will be fun to be in charge, but it's also a playful way to let your partner know about all those not-so-obvious hot spots of yours.

FRANTASTIC FRANGELICO

There's nothing quite like a little Frangelico to cleanse the palate and sweeten the sex. A sweet, hazelnut liqueur, Frangelico tingles the tongue and warms the body. . . . So just imagine the possibilities. Pour a glass, savor a sip, and make out passionately with your lover until the tingles wear off. Then take another sip and repeat. Now get ready to have a little more fun with it. Dab a drop of Frangelico on his nipples, on her belly button—think of all the hot spots. Now lick it off, suck it up . . . and you know what comes next. Warm and tingly, here we come!

POPSICLE PERFECTION

What better way to head out of the realm of sex foods and into sex toys. Popsicles are amazing sex toys—and they're always available right in your local grocery store. There are so many ways to enjoy them—for him and her. So always keep a box in the freezer.

Strip him, tell him to lie down, and blindfold him (blocking one of his senses to heighten the rest). Now get ready. You can get totally naked, too, but you don't have to. Just make sure you're wearing something sexy. Straddle him as you savor your favorite flavor of Popsicle. Hum as you lick and suck it, and as it melts, let it drip and splatter on him. But be sure to lap up the drops before they dry. Where you drip is where you lick, so have some fun with it as it drips onto his

Naughty Nibble

Drinking and sex can be a great combination. A 1994 study published in the journal *Nature* says alcohol raises women's levels of testosterone, a hormone linked to libido in both sexes. Not to mention how a glass of wine can relax inhibitions. Just don't overdo it. What a waste of a night if you're too drunk to feel anything and actually enjoy yourself.

lips, his neck, his nipples, his tummy, his . . . You get the idea.

To pleasure her with a Popsicle, she must also be naked, lying down, and blindfolded—why not, right? Have your favorite-flavor Popsicle nearby. With the tip of the Popsicle, trace small circles all over her body—her wrists and inner arms, her shoulders and neck, her nipples and tummy . . . You get the idea. As you create your circles, follow the trail and lap up the juice with the tip of your tongue. The sensations of cold and hard from the Popsicle followed by the warm and smooth sensations of your tongue will drive her wild.

How kinky are you feeling now? Kinky enough to use that Popsicle like a dildo? If you're not, don't worry. You've already taken kinky to a new level. But if you are, then you and your partner are both in for a treat. Slip a condom on the Popsicle (you don't want her to end up with a yeast infection), and alternating between the Popsicle and your tongue, go down on your lover, driving her wild with the sensations of hot and cold. Lick around her labia and clit as you penetrate her with the Popsicle. Now, that's kinky.

NOW YOU KNOW . . .

There are so many inventive, delicious ways to savor and enjoy your favorite foods, and create erotic associations to last a lifetime. In the next chapter, we'll move on to using sex toys, edible and not, and the many loving and inventive ways there are to pleasure your partner with plastic and other materials. Can you handle the kink? Turn the page and see.

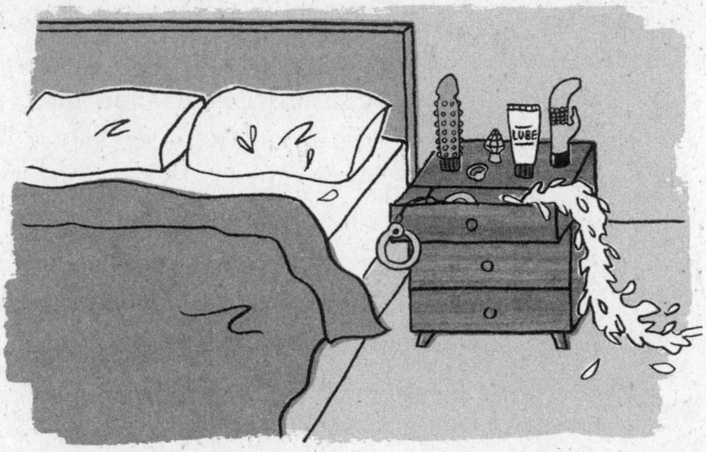

Chapter 7

Vrrrroom. Whirrrrr. Ahhhh.

Does it get any kinkier than sex toys? Well, actually, yes . . . but we have the whole second half of the book to explore such things. For now, when it comes to leaving the sensually safe realm of the tried and trusted and somewhat tame, sex toys are definitely a great place to start.

You may have heard of vibrators and dildos and butt plugs and other assorted toys—and maybe you've already experimented with some or even all of these. But no matter what experience you've already had, you're guaranteed to find something in this chapter kinky enough to make you look at your sex toys—and other items in your house, for that matter—with a whole new kinky perspective.

Keep in mind that not all sex toys require batteries—and not all are made from plastic or other synthetic materials. In fact, you may be surprised at just how many "sex toys" you already have lying around (remember the Popsicles in the last chapter?). We'll look at these first, then move into some of the most fun adult toys and novelties available.

Naughty Nibble

Sometimes sex toys make a partner feel insecure, that he or she may be inadequate and hence the need for a sexual aid. But you can put those fears aside with a little love and reassurance, and a whole lot of playful experimentation.

There are plenty of adult-entertainment stores you can access online or via mail, many featured in the Resources section of this book, who will handle your business with respect and discretion. Pursue the offerings on your own at first if that makes you more comfortable, but then get your partner involved. Glance through the selection of toys as well as various props, massage oils, videos, and so forth. Open up a dialogue with your partner about the items you see, and let your partner know what interests you—and encourage your partner to do the same. Order a few things, and when the package arrives, it will be like Christmas morning in your bedroom—no matter what the time of year.

A TRUE MASTERPIECE

We learned in the last chapter that body painting is a wonderful way to play with your partner's body. In addition to chocolate, body paint and brushes make excellent toys. Washable, nontoxic, and even edible kits can be found at sex stores or over the Internet—and there are even glow-in-the-dark varieties. (See Resources.)

Take turns making each other into erotic masterpieces. Maybe write an erotic love fantasy on his or her back that can be fulfilled only if guessed, or label what you consider your partner's "hot spots" from 1 to 10—the nape of her neck, maybe the back of his knees, his or her nipples. If you guess right, you get rewarded by actually pleasuring that spot on your partner. But even if you guess wrong, you've just found a fun, comfortable forum for your partner to communicate to you what he or she truly desires and needs. Everybody wins.

SALAD DAYS

We talked a lot about using food in a sensual manner in the last chapter, but food also plays a significant role in the sex-toy world. And the produce section of your local grocery store is just chockfull of naughty notions. Like the cucumber—Nature's dildo. In size and texture, it resembles a man's manhood (if sometimes slightly exaggerated in size). And then there's the durability factor. What other vegetable can withstand such rigorous prodding so well? Interesting alternates to cucumbers include carrots, for a more, well, streamlined experience, and celery, which, because of its shape, procures a special kind of pleasure.

FRUIT COCK-TAIL

What kind of dirty thoughts pop into your head when you see a nice big bowl of ice-cold blueberries? True, they're a bit too small to be used as Ben Wa balls (small metal balls, sometimes tied together, that are inserted into the vagina to cause sexual stimulation for a woman when she walks or moves her

thighs), but what if he places them around—or even inside—
her special parts and eats them out? The cold from the blueberries, the warmth of his tongue . . . Need more be said?

In the last chapter, we explored the erotic prowess of a
regular, everyday, usually innocent little orange. With this
idea of "male stimulation" in mind, what are some other
fruits you could try? A grapefruit? A tomato? What about
using two peeled bananas—one on either side on his shaft—
smushing them into his skin as you stimulate, and giving his
member the sexy sensation of being someplace soft and
sweet and slippery?

Really use your imagination here, but whatever you do,
please be sure that any produce you use is clean before it
nears any points of entry. Even better, slip a condom on your
carrot or cucumber or zucchini squash, because there's nothing sexy about getting an infection. Whatever fruits or vegetables you choose to defile, grocery shopping will probably
never seem like such a chore ever again.

KITCHEN AIDS

Look around your kitchen for a minute. What do you see?
Your kitchen is full of erotic possibilities—and not just in
the refrigerator. It's a veritable treasure trove of sex toys just
begging to be discovered.

Are you into spanking? We'll get more into this in Chapter 8, but there are many devices right there in your kitchen
that you can use to give your partner a playful pat. A spatula
(a rubber one—no metal, please), for example, is a great tool
for spanking, as is a wooden spoon. Hold it between your
fingers (not in your fist) to ensure that there won't be too
much power behind your pat and lightly tap your partner on

the tush. (Note: To figure out how hard to pat, test on a scale from 1 to 5, with 1 as the softest and 5 as hardest. As you play, ask your partner what number they want, and as long as you're not involved in a heated domination game, allow your partner to call out and change the number as you spank.) If your partner has been especially "naughty," you might try one of those handheld spatter screens (the ones that look like small tennis rackets).

If you're into cupping—that is, you enjoy actually cupping the breasts, testicles, or other parts of the body—a large metal serving spoon is a wonderful device. Use it as is or run it under cold water for cooling or hot for a warming sensation. Ooo la la.

Even those clips you use to close bags of chips can be dirty when called into service as nipple clamps. Traditionally, nipple clamps are made from metal and come in either a clover clamp or tweezer clamp style. But they don't have to be, which is why the chip clips, made of plastic and designed to hold not too tight, can be great starter clamps. The thrill comes in the pressure applied and getting the balance between pain and pleasure just right.

Now take another look around the kitchen. What can you come up with?

> ## Just for Her . . .
>
> Sometimes men become overwhelmed by all they think they're *supposed* to do to sexually satisfy women. So, ladies, sometimes it's okay to *just do it*—without any planning or staging or drama. Just give in to sweet spontaneity and enjoy.

NOT IN VAIN

Move through the rest of your home and what do you see? What other innocent household items can be repurposed to a sexier use? Look on the top of her vanity table. An everyday hairbrush is a great sex toy for spanking, and one of those large makeup brushes makes for a great tickler. Start training yourself to see the sexual potential of any household item and you'll never run out of possibilities.

PILLOW PERFECTION

Pillows make excellent sex toys when used as "props." In the doggie-style position, place pillows lengthwise from her breasts to her pelvis to help make her more comfortable. In missionary, place a pillow under the lower half of her back, which tilts her pelvis forward. This is a great way for her to achieve a G-spot orgasm in this position. And note: He should not get too fixated on "aiming for her belly button" here. At this angle, every thrust will stimulate and massage the G-spot—and there's no way you can miss it using this technique.

THREE SHEETS TO THE WIND

Sheets as sex toys? You bet. And the higher the thread count, the better. As restraints, typical bedsheets are soft and not scary, like, say, leather straps or handcuffs or more hard-core-type restraints. Tie up just your lover's wrists—to each other or to the bed—for a light thrill. And if you're looking for a little more control, tie up your partner's legs as well. We'll get more into playful bondage a bit later, but this is definitely a safe, nonthreatening way to introduce it into your lovemaking.

Naughty Nibble

Invest in some high-thread-count silky or satin sheets, but don't tell your partner about it. Put them on the bed without him knowing and wait for the look of pleasure and surprise on his face when he slips into bed that night. What a luxurious stage for your next show of amour.

THOSE NAUGHTY NOVELTIES

Party stores can spur the imagination. One of my favorite tricks is to buy the funky buttons that light up and flash and sometimes vibrate. Ladies, tell him to expect a surprise at dinner tonight. Turn down all the lights and pin the party lights to your underwear and bra and serve him dinner this way. It's not overtly sexual, but it will definitely draw his attention to those delights he'd like to see on the dinner menu any night.

DESSERT TRAY

Break out one of the nice trays you received as a wedding gift and never used, and arrange on it an assortment of several sexy items—oil, chocolate kisses, flavored lubricants, and various sex toys. Bring it into the bedroom and think of all the sexy ways you can tease and tantalize your partner with all your sexy selections. When you get to him, you can let him choose what he'd like to play with, or you can decide for him—whatever the mood calls for.

ROCK YOUR WORLD

As we've seen, a sex toy does not require a motor or batteries to be effective. It's what you bring to it—how you repurpose it—that makes all the difference. Moving throughout your home, the possibilities should just be popping out right about now. But don't limit your thinking to small objects. Furniture can also make for some really cool sex toys. For instance, do you have a rocking chair? If not, invest in one. A rocking chair can become quite a spectacular sex toy—but it has to be big enough for the both of you to rock in. Here's how:

He sits down first and invites her to sit on his lap, facing him. And if this isn't obvious already, you should both be naked. Now he pulls up his penis so it sits between her legs and holds it firmly up against her—but no entering yet. Now start rocking back and forth, getting comfy with the motion and closeness you feel all pressed up against each other. As you rock, he should begin rubbing his shaft up and down the outside of her love mound. When it feels like climax is coming, let him in. Keep rocking as the sexual tension builds and the excitement rushes you all the way to totally rocking your worlds.

LEI DAY

You don't always have to be blatant to be kinky. If you're in the mood for sex, why not have a little fun with double meanings? Head to a party store and purchase a bunch of Hawaiian-style leis. Let your partner know that you're planning a luau for the end of the day, and let her know where and when she is expected. When she arrives, be sure you are wearing a lei around your neck. And nothing else. Then enjoy the feast. Talk about getting leid . . . After the fact, wear one of the other leis you purchased every time you're in the mood as a subtle—or maybe not-so-subtle—hint that you have more on your mind than where to take your next vacation.

UNDER ARREST

Purchase a pair of furry handcuffs from a sex-toy catalog on your own and leave them somewhere your partner will notice them (though nowhere that your kids can). When he finds them and asks you what they're for, tell him they're for *you*—that you'd like your partner to handcuff you to the bed and make love to you. To make it even more exciting, tell your partner that it's always been a big fantasy for you and that tonight's the night.

BOY BUZZ

Many men quite mistakenly believe that vibrators are strictly for their partners' pleasure. It's time to prove the men wrong. Ladies, break out your trusted friend and treat your man to an experience he won't ever forget. Take your vibrator and tease him with it around his crotch area. If he responds, stimulate some of his other sensitive areas, like his nipples. Break out some of your favorite massage oil, rub it into his skin, and vibe him again. Playfully tease his less obvious hot spots before getting to the main event.

Once you're there, gently, playfully vibe around the base of his penis and his testicles. And don't forget the perineum—the space between his testicles and tush. You can indirectly stimulate this male version of the G-spot, sometimes called the "P-spot," if you vibe him at the section closer to the anus.

You can prolong the ecstasy by taking a "make-out break." As he gets closer to climax, move away from his lower regions and turn your focus to his face. Stroke and kiss him. Really love him. Now go back to stim-

Just for Him . . .

Vibrators aren't just for the ladies. Your wife or girlfriend can show you what all the buzz is about and give you an explosive orgasm with a vibrator—if you just ask. One suggestion is that the next time she goes down on you, have her rest the vibrator against her cheek while she's at it. The vibe will indirectly vibrate your penis and give you an insanely intense orgasm.

ulating him. He should be going nuts by now, so just get the man off.

BUZZ THRILL

You've heard the term "buzz kill." That's about as far from accurate as this next trick could be. Guys, invest in a small vibe called a Turbo Bullet (see Resources) and pull it out while you're going down on your partner. Turn it on and clench it between your lips, tracing her sensitive parts with the tip of the bullet. Now, as you pleasure her, wherever your tongue goes, the toy follows.

WATER LILY

A famous Hollywood party girl taught me this trick, which requires a waterproof vibrator, a penchant for prolonging passion, and, as always, lots of love.

After your kids are in bed, plan to take a shower with your partner and one of these gadgets. Enjoy soaping each other up, massaging, kissing, fondling. Now, guys, go down on your lover, using your tongue on one side of her sensitive region while using the waterproof vibrator on the other side. Get her all riled up, then take a break. Use the vibrator on her breasts, stimulating all around and saving the nipples for last. Now head south again—and back and forth between here and her breasts. Then stop. Then

Abracadabra

They don't call the Hitachi vibrator the "Magic Wand" for nothing. With two speeds, it's one of the oldest toys on the market and, as it plugs right into the wall, you never have to worry about batteries. Women can use it on their own, but it's also a lot of fun to use with a partner, especially during intercourse. The size and shape make it almost impossible not to climax—no matter what position you're in. For instance, while you're in doggie style, the head of the toy can be placed on or near her clitoris while he takes her. For best results, set it to low and let the orgasm really build. For best results in the missionary position, he needs to be positioned a little off center when he enters and thrusts so he doesn't inadvertently knock it out of the way with his tummy.

And even if she is using it on her own, she can share the experience and make it even better. While she lies on her back and pleasures herself with the wand, he can get involved, kissing her neck and breasts, rubbing small circles on her tummy, whatever feels good.

start again. After several times of this back-and-forth, combined with the steam of the shower and the heat of the water, she's guaranteed to have a massive O. (Check out the Resources section to learn where to purchase one of these water babies.)

BULLETED POINTS

The Bullet vibrator is one of my absolute favorites. Most are small, and because of their size, they're also easy to control. Tease her with it, circling around her clitoris and only occasionally grazing the top. When she gets super-excited, stop.

Naughty Nibble

Vibrators come in all kinds of shapes and sizes. There are ones that are egg-shaped, bullet-shaped, penis-shaped (like the Rabbit, see page 127), ones that fit over your finger, ones that attach to a belt she can drape over her clitoris. The possibilities are limitless, and there truly is something for everyone.

Go down on her for a while and then alternate the toy with your tongue. Getting her to peak, and alternating the stimulation, makes for a powerful orgasm.

And a Bullet isn't just for her. He can learn to love this portable pleasure device just as much as she. Slip a small bullet into a condom, turn it on low, and tease his perineum with it. Some men will be open to anal play with a vibrator, but some will not. Don't press the issue. If he's open to trying it out, be sure to use plenty of lube and gently insert just the very tip of the Bullet. Let him savor the sensation of the vibration for a while, and insert more if he's up for it. Just be careful you don't insert it so much that you can't take it out.

THE MAGIC FINGER

Vibrators that fit on your finger give you lots of flexibility and they're pretty unobtrusive. You know how good it feels to have your lover glide his or her fingertips over you, just grazing the surface of your skin? Now imagine how electrifying this sensation becomes with a vibrator that slips onto your fingertip.

For her or him, use the finger vibrator to stimulate arms and shoulders, neck and chest. Lightly graze the nipples, the tummy, the line that runs between the navel and the lower regions. Run your vibrating finger along your partner's feet and legs, and up and down their inner thighs. When your partner reaches the threshold of the point of no return, push him or her over the edge. For her, circle around her clitoris and enter her. Leave the tip of your finger vibrating right on her G-spot as you delicately kiss her face and neck. For him, graze his perineum and testicles with the vibe as you gently lick and kiss his shaft. And then take him home.

> **Naughty Nibble**
>
> Choose a vibrator with adjustable speeds so you can more easily orchestrate the many sensations.

HOPPIN' HAPPY

Ever since *Sex and the City* made them popular, everybody's gotta have a Rabbit. And that's a very good thing. A bit more intense than your standard vibrator, Rabbits come in various shapes, including ones that look just like penises (I mean, gigantic ones in a rainbow of colors). It is designed to swerve in several directions at once, as well as to vibrate and even pulse. But the reason it's called a Rabbit is its "ears." The top of the Rabbit has two, designed to sit right on her clitoris (or her anus, depending on which way you hold it—and what will give her the most pleasure) as the shaft part is inserted inside of her.

YOURS, MINE, AND OURS

Dual vibes offer good vibrations for him and her. When using these, start off facing each other, each partner stimulating him- or herself. Now switch and begin stimulating each other. Now continue going back and forth like this for as long as you can possibly stand it.

> **Naughty Nibble**
>
> Here are a few of my all-time-favorite sex toys: the Pocket Rocket, the Turbo Magnum Vibrating Bullet, the Rabbit, and the Motif Vibe. See Resources to find out how to make them yours.

FOR HIS PLEASURE...

A lot of men complain that sex toys are mainly for women, but there are many designed just for men—and many ways to pleasure a man even with the ones designed for women. All it takes is a little creativity, a little sensitivity in knowing what your partner will like—and a well-honed sense of adventure for both partners.

Here's one trick women can use on their men that's guaranteed to make them insane with pleasure. Place a small washcloth in the dryer to heat it to warm—but not too hot. Now place it over his package while he lies on his back. Next, take a small vibrator, like the Pocket Rocket (see Resources), and turn it on low. Roll it over the towel, experimenting with different speeds and directions. The towel actually spreads the vibration all throughout the genital area and feels heavenly. What a way to relax.

JELLY-LICIOUS

There is a jellylike tube that fits over the penis and that can he can use on his own or she can use on him for the hand job of his life. Here's how it works: Pour Astroglide or another water-based lube to coat the inside of the cylinder. Now stretch the device to fit around his manhood and begin squeezing and sliding it up and down. Get creative with your movements. Instead of a steady "up and down," break it up with a swirling motion every few strokes. Whatever feels good, of course.

Just for Her...

Girls, if you want great orgasms, you have to get those sex muscles toned and tight. Start today. You can do your Kegels and you can also invest in a pair of vaginal barbells. No, I'm not kidding. Available through most adult stores, these will give you strength training like you've never experienced before. (See Resources.)

LORD OF THE RING

Rings made to wear around the penis are called "cock rings" and are generally made of rubber and quite pliable. They're used to help a man maintain an erection by restricting blood flow. As soon as he "stands at attention," the ring is fastened at the base of his penis, behind the testicles. It's a great time for her to take charge and show him who's boss, with everything under her control.

OH, SWEET SUCTION...

There's a toy available for women that's a suction device that fits right over the vulva. When you turn it on, it creates suction, which draws the blood to that area, making her hypersensitive. After five to ten minutes of stimulation, indulge in intercourse and see if it doesn't make both partners more orgasmic—her because of the increased blood flow, and him because she is more engorged and therefore feels softer and plumper, like a soft, sexy, satisfyingly squishy cushion.

DILDO DREAMS

Dildos have been used in sexplay since the beginning of time, and there's definitely a dildo available to suit any taste, with tons of variation in length, girth, color, and even material—though most people swear by silicone. Why? They are super-high-quality, nonporous, and easy to keep clean. If you are allergic to silicone, slap a condom on it.

Naughty Nibble

Did you know there are kits available that you can use to clone your or your partner's special parts for a customized sex toy? Head to www.cloneyourbone .com for his; www .matchyoursnatch.com for hers.

Naughty Nibble

The G-Spot Positioning Strap (also known as the Doggie-Style Enhancing Strap) is excellent for G-spot stimulation and also makes rear entry much more comfortable and satisfying for her. See Resources for sex stores.

Most couples will use a dildo on her, but there are some adventurous men who may be willing to try it out. Whatever you do, don't forget the lube. And be sure to keep it clean—the dildo, that is. The *action* itself should be dirty with a capital *D*.

THIS DOESN'T SUCK (WELL, TECHNICALLY, IT DOES)

This type of dildo is definitely for only the most kinky. The dildo itself doesn't offer any suction action, but it has a suction cup at the end that you can attach to a mirror, to the floor so you can straddle it, or to somewhere "hip high." Then you invite your man to his very own sex show. Turn off the lights. Light some candles and do your dildo. Trust me, he will freak. With the mirror there you can see all kinds of hotness, and he'll learn how you like your thrusts. Tell him when he's had enough of the show to let you know and he can be next up.

AND SPEAKING OF SUCK . . .

Dildos and oral sex are a marriage made in heaven. What works best is when the dildo used actually resembles his penis, so be sure to purchase one that isn't too far off from the real thing.

Now, men, slowly penetrate your lover just a tiny bit—not more than an inch—with the tip of the dildo. Slowly massage the wall of her vagina, going deeper and deeper but never more than a couple of inches. After a good ten min-

Fun with Fetishes: Sensory Sensuality

Fetishes can be experienced and enjoyed with all your senses. Here are some common ways.

Sight: Color Fetish

Some people get turned on by colors. Are you or your partner among them? Experiment by wearing various colors and see if anything turns you or your partner on. If you hit on one that gets your partner's attention, try to don it as often as possible—whether that means special lingerie or boxers, or even wearing shirts in that color around your partner.

Smell: Scent Fetish

It's a little known fact that many men get turned on by the scent of pumpkin. Others, men and women, have been known to get turned on by the scent of chocolate-chip cookies baking. Next time you're feeling amorous, why not bake something special for your beloved and see what happens.

Feel: Buried in Sand Fetish

If you don't have a beach nearby, you'll have to save this for a vacation. And yes, it's messy, but just try it. Your partner lies down on their back in the sand and you cover their whole body except their face. This works better if the sand is a little wet, but try it both ways, with wet sand or with dry.

Sound: Listening to Sexy Sounds Fetish

Some people get more turned on by what they hear than what they see. Does that describe your partner or you? You can find out by

(continued on next page)

watching a porn DVD that features a lot of vocalizing. Either close your eyes or have your partner blindfold you (or the other way around) as you listen to all the "Ooohs" and "Aaahs" and "Oh Gods."

Taste: Fun with Food

See Chapter 6.

utes of this teasing, start going down on her while you continue to manipulate your silicone clone. Control your movements—as excited as you get, don't thrust too hard. Keep the same gentle pace as you pleasure her and she'll be well on her way to orgasm heaven.

TWO'S COMPANY–THREE'S A PARTY

If you and your partner ever fantasized about having a threesome and don't feel comfortable bringing another player into your sexplay, you can have a wonderful make-believe threesome with your new friend, Dildo. This time, you want to pick up a dildo that doesn't resemble you in any way—to keep the fantasy alive.

The next time you make love, start off with him entering. Then pull out and switch to the dildo. Use the dildo for a couple of minutes, then go back to him. And then alternate again. If both partners are feeling especially kinky, you may opt to lube up the dildo and insert it in her anus or vagina while you place your penis in her mouth. Or, for the kinkiest of the kinky, insert your penis in her while doggie style, and insert the dildo in her anus at the same time. We'll get more into these forbidden pleasures in the last chapter.

DILDO MARKS THE SPOT

A G-spot dildo is specially designed for just that—for hitting the G-spot upon entry. (See Resources.) Insert the dildo and place the tip of the toy right on her G-spot. Manipulate the dildo to massage her G-spot a good ten minutes at least. Now take your hand and massage her lower abdomen while you're manipulating the dildo, trying to connect the inner G-spot stimulation with the outer.

Just for Her . . .

Dim the lights and draw the curtains. It's time to put on a show for your man. And here's the catch: No matter how turned on he gets, he's not allowed to touch you till morning.

While you're getting ready for bed tonight, strut around wearing nothing but a long, silk scarf or a boa, with a vibrator or dildo in your hand. Put on some sexy music and dance around for him. Place the sex toy down next to him and really work what you got with the scarf or boa, slowly gliding it around your body in as sensual a manner as possible. Now lie on your back and glide the scarf up and down on your lower regions as you stroke and fondle your nipples and breasts.

Now jump up unexpectedly and grab your sex toy. Give it a nice lube, whether with a bottled lubricant or, even better for him, with your mouth. As you play with your toy, be sure you, um, face him so he gets to see every detail, every thrust. Now enjoy getting yourself off and the feeling of power it gives you.

Sample Sale

There are sex toys specifically designed for women and for men, but as far as I'm concerned, most can be used to pleasure both—and in so many wonderful ways.

Bullets and **Eggs** are excellent for clitoral stimulation. **Bnaughty** is waterproof, has multiple speeds, and is my personal favorite bullet, and **Cyberflicker** is my favorite egg.

My First Vibe and **Slimline** are basic cylindrical vibes. Many first-timers start here and use it for vaginal and anal stimulation and penetration. The sizes vary, and when possible always get the option for variable-speed vibration.

Realistics look like penises and are good for penetration and fantasy.

The **Jolie: Intense Clitoral Pleasure** is 100 percent waterproof (so it can be used in the bathtub), it's compact, but it packs a punch!

The **Libertie** has three speeds and is excellent for G-spot stimulation.

The **Ideal** is similar to the Hitachi Magic Wand (see page 125), but it's smaller—which means more flexibility in terms of sex positions.

Mini massagers like the **Pocket Rocket** are great for clitoral stimulation and small enough to fit in your purse

Crystal Wand, Nubby G Vibe, and **G-Whiz** are all excellent G-spot stimulators.

Fantasy Fingers, Finger Fun, Fukuoku 9000 are my favorite finger vibes.

Laya Spot works great for clitoral stimulation.

SaSi Vibrator is my latest discovery—and it's amazing! Contoured and smooth, it vibrates softly, and the movement type, speed, and vibration are all adjustable. But that's not the best part.

SaSi has "sensual intelligence," which means you can program it to remember your favorite speed and movement.

The **Rock Chick** is a U-shaped toy with a hooked end for G-spot stimulation and a wider, ridged end for clitoral and labia stimulation. You use it by rocking the toy forward and back, which nudges the G-spot and rubs the clitoris at the same time.

PLUG THIS

For adventurous folks who like a little buttplay (and we'll get into this much more in Chapter 11), a butt plug is a truly exciting device. They come in all sizes and shapes, with textures designed for maximum tush titillation. Use it simply to stimulate the anus or, with lots of lube and love, to penetrate. The key here is to start small and always go slowly. And if one partner calls it quits, it's over.

NOW YOU KNOW . . .

Adult toys can be as mild and innocent as fruits and vegetables—and run the gamut all the way to the naughtiest of naughty. There's something for every erotic taste. And the use of sex toys does not mean one partner is lacking—in fact, far from it. If anything, introducing toys into your sexplay only shows how resourceful, open, and imaginative you are.

And speaking of imagination . . . We're about to enter the most imaginative section of the kinky realm: fantasy and role-playing. So lock your inhibitions in the closet and get ready to focus on fabulous fulfillment.

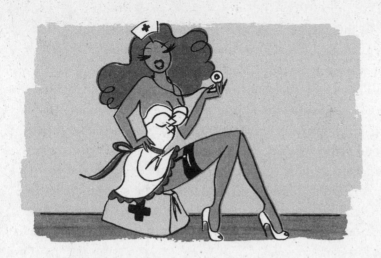

Chapter 8

Fun with Fantasy and Role-Play

There are few sexual things that test the limits of your inhibitions and the comfort level of yourself and your partner as role-play. This type of exercise not only forces you to open up to expressing yourself in new and exciting physical ways, it also challenges you to be vulnerable and, therefore, trusting with your partner. You're both in on the game and there are no judgments made—even in the most hilariously awkward moments.

This chapter isn't just about donning a costume and pretending to be someone else for a new sexual thrill. It's about pure fantasy and all that entails. So while it could mean taking a trip to the costume store to pick out sexy nurse and doctor outfits, it's also about what happens on the trip. . . . Say, if you decided to dress up in character and pull over and enjoy a secret tryst in a private—or not so private—spot on the way back from the store.

In this chapter, I will not only give you some fun scenarios to enact, I'll also give you some delightful, inspiring ways to fuel your fantasies. It's all about kinky, right?

The most important thing is to think of this chapter as a launchpad to fuel your most frisky fantasies. What I have here are suggestions intended to spark you to start thinking about some of your wildest dirty dreams . . . but I'm not going to dictate to you what makes you hot and bothered. So as you read through these suggestions, be sure to do so together. Talk about what excites you or repulses you about each, and tailor them to your taste. I can get you started, but the rest is up to you.

OH, RACY ROMANCE

A safe, tame way to begin exploring some of your fantasies together is through the written word. Hey, they're called "bodice rippers" for a reason: Romance novels are packed with white-hot passages of passionate lust, with dashing men so driven to possess beautiful women, they'll tear the heroine's clothes right off to get to the luscious lady flesh. Suffice to say, the sex scenes can get pretty steamy and are thus great inspiration for role-play.

If you haven't read a romance novel before—I'm talking to the girls and guys here—why not give it a whirl? Try books by Anne Stuart for intense, graphic sex. Stephanie Laurens, Madeline Hunter, and Sophie Jordan all heat up the historical romance genre, while books by Jeaniene Frost put the "porn" in paranormal. And if it's a contemporary setting that amps your amour, Linda Howard and Lori Foster really know how to thrill. And the best part of all this? You can buy these books right in the grocery store. While you're reading, just be sure to highlight the passages that make you really hot so you can share them with your partner.

WORDS INTO ACTION

Speaking of highlighting scenes in your favorite romance novels . . . What better time to share these scenes than in bed? Give your lover the basic plot of your new novel and read some of the sex scenes you've highlighted aloud. Let your partner know how these scenes echo your own secret fantasies, and invite your partner to act one out with you. And if that goes over well, why not make up some of your own together?

> ## Just for Her . . .
> Certain words are sex triggers for men, so find out which ones light your guy's fire and use them anytime you're feeling horny. He'll get the point.

A FEMME FORUM

Many men's magazines are targeted to trigger the sexual desires of men. Look at a nudie magazine and you'll see lots of graphic visuals that, depending on the magazine, can be a little much for most women to bear. But they aren't all like that. Magazines like *Playboy* and *Penthouse* are artfully photographed and also feature a fair amount of actual "content."

Penthouse, for instance, has plenty of titillating photos, but it also features the famed "Forum" section, in which readers relay their "real" sexual experiences. And they're actually a lot of fun to read. In the spirit of reading aloud from erotic novels, try sharing some of these letters with each other tonight. Scan through and find one that really sets you a-tingle and read it out loud. What about this passage really excites you? What are some of the situations he wishes he could find himself in? Not only will it open your sexual mind, you'll get to know something more about your partner's sexuality, and you may even spark a new experience for you to share.

ADVISE YOUR PLAYBOY

Playboy also has a letters section you can use to learn more about each other: the "Advisor." Why not explore it together? Tonight, after the kids are asleep, run a nice warm bath and get cozy together in it with your magazine. First flip through together and talk about how you feel about the pictures. When you get to the "Advisor" section, read some of the letters out loud. Ask your lover how he or she would have answered some of the letters and share how you would have. Not only does this get the dirty parts of your brain revved up and ready for fantasy, it shows your partner that you're open to talking turn-ons, as well as giving some of his or hers a whirl.

DRESS ME UP, DRESS ME DOWN

Ever notice, when you're all dressed up and looking spiffy, that you each seem to have a newfound interest in the other? Of course you do—you look hot when you're not wearing your dirty old baseball cap or your "mom jeans."

Okay, so you've been stuck at home with young kids and don't have a lot of opportunities to go to fancy places. But who says you have to go anywhere at all when you get all decked out? Tonight, why not don your best duds and hang out together in your bedroom. Plan a Bedroom Banquet (see page 106) or just enjoy a bottle of champagne. Whatever you choose, keep in mind that one of the supreme highlights of dressing up this way is the moment each of you undresses the other. . . .

THESE BOOTS ARE MADE FOR . . .

What woman doesn't feel sexy and empowered by Nancy Sinatra's signature number, "These Boots Are Made for Walking"? Now you can make it your signature *bedroom* number—as you explore all the ways a sexy pair of boots are made for anything but taking a walk.

Tonight, load this song into the CD player in your bedroom and slip into a pair of your sexiest boots. If you don't have a pair of sexy boots, go out and get them. And the higher the better—meaning both the boot and the heel. Before bed, play the song and start prancing around wearing nothing but your sexy boots. When he asks what's gotten into you, tell him you've always wanted to make love with your boots on. And tonight's the night.

LOVELY LATEX

This might be totally out of character, but that's all the more reason you should do it. It's good to break out and be somebody different for a change. Latex is hot in all of its forms,

Fun with Fetishes: Fashion

In Chapter 6, we got a taste of some favorite food fetishes, but clothing fetishes are probably the most common fetishes of all—fixations on everything from corsets to uniforms, from leather to lingerie, and on and on. Sometimes the object is absolutely necessary for sexual arousal and sometimes it's just a light, fun addition. Here are some of the top ones:

Underwear Fetishes

These are really popular and go both ways—meaning you can really enjoy doing all kinds of things with underwear, or you really like the idea of no undies at all. For those who love it, putting yours or your lover's undies in the freezer for ten minutes is sure to create all kinds of good chills. For those who like to go without, on your next date night, neither of you are to wear underwear. Just be sure you spend the evening reminding each other about it.

Black Dress Fetish

Ladies, make a pact with your man that every time you wear a black dress, it means you're looking for action. Now start collecting them—especially ones that are form-fitting and low-cut to expose lots of luscious cleavage. (Note: You can also do the same with a collection of short skirts.)

Lingerie Fetish

This one is so common, it's almost cliché. But that doesn't mean it can't be fun! On your next date night, she should wear an outfit that will reveal one piece of sexy lingerie under her clothes. When you get home, she then slips into something entirely different. And once that piece of lingerie gets torn off and thrown to the floor, she can put on another hot piece to sleep in. Or maybe not sleep right away . . .

Leather Fetish

This one comes up a lot in bondage scenarios (see Chapter 9). If you don't feel like donning a full-on leather outfit, you don't have to. Start small, wearing a leather collar, bracelet, top, or undies.

Fur Fetish

Many people, myself included, love the feeling of making love on fur. Why not purchase a fake animal-fur throw blanket, toss it in front of the fireplace, strip down, and invite your partner to join you for some "animal" action.

and it's time you invested in some. All the sex-toy stores and many lingerie stores carry latex bra-and-panty sets, dresses, bodysuits, and yes, even stuff for the guys.

There's something about latex and skin that seems so bad, so be bad, really bad. Surprise your partner with your new kinky couture by greeting him or her at the door when he or she comes home at night, wearing your bathrobe over your "outfit." Escort your partner to the bedroom and drop the robe, asking what he or she thinks of your slippery new threads. Tell your honey how much you want to be with him or her and how you've been thinking about him all day. Then kiss your lover passionately until neither one of you can take it anymore. Do you leave the latex on or take it off? Well, that's for the two of you to decide.

SUPERFREAK

"She's a very kinky girl, the kind you don't take home to mother. . . ." Rick James made the concept of kinky super-cool, and this legendary song can go a long way in setting the mood for a blissfully kinky romp. Once you do it to this song, thrusting and pulsating your pelvis to the beat, it can become a special, subtle signal to your partner. From that first time on, every time you want to get your freak on, just press play.

THE PICKUP ARTIST

In the very beginning of the movie *When a Man Loves a Woman*, Meg Ryan is sitting at a bar when she's approached by Andy Garcia. They make some small talk and, much to the shock of those around them, especially the other guys for whom she was playing "hard to get," she almost immediately agrees to go back to his place. Then we find out that they are actually married, mortgaged, and have children. But despite all this (and her drinking problem, which threatens to tear them apart), they still like to keep it kinky. And what a quick, easy way to reignite the old passion—by pretending to be strangers again.

For your next date night, leave your wedding rings at home (if you can) and arrange to meet separately at a bar—or even a park, a bookstore, or the zoo. It doesn't really matter where. When you finally meet, pretend you don't know each other. What would be especially fun is if one of you were flirting with someone else at the time you do come together. Then the other can swoop in, lay on the charm, and claim their prize. Where you take it next is entirely up to you!

ME TARZAN, YOU JANE

She's a lady shipwrecked on a deserted island, the only sur-vivor of an ocean liner that met a terrible fate. He's a savage jungle man, prancing around in a loincloth (oh heck, this isn't Hollywood—it's more like he's naked as can be). He grunts his wants—and she's at the top of the list. She can't make out what he's saying, but she understands the message: "You my plaything. You satisfy me, I keep you safe from the lions and tigers and other savages on the island." He has no mores or social graces—he's an animal who lives by his urges and takes what he wants whenever he wants it. And she, raised in a proper, civilized household without so much as a cat or a dog around, must give up everything she's learned as she, too, indulges all her most primal urges.

HOT FOR TEACHER

Are you ready for some serious role-playing now? This one can be tailored to put either partner in the teacher's seat, but here we'll put her in the position of authority, with him as the naughty student needing her special brand of disci-pline.

So, ladies, find yourself a nerdy pair of glasses and a con-servative suit. Make it something "marmish," like what an old-fashioned schoolteacher might wear—but be sure to wear very sexy undergarments underneath. If you can, tie up your hair in a bun and slip on a pair of sexy high heels. You want to provide some clue to get him thinking.

Ask him to sit down, telling him you need to teach him a lesson about satisfying a woman, and, without cracking yourself up too much, tell him this is a very serious situation and if he doesn't take it seriously, you will need to discipline him accordingly.

Now hand him a paper and pen and tell him to draw a naked woman. Take his silly drawing and, with a red pen, mark all your favorite hot spots and tell him why they are so hot. Let him know where and when you like these spots to be touched, and when you get finished marking them all, take down your hair, pull off your suit, and show him the real thing. Just be firm with him, letting him know that he's not allowed to touch anything until you've shown him *all* your hot zones. By the time you get to the last one, he'll be practically leaping from his seat with lust.

BOND GIRL

Bond Girls are famous for their sultry, sexy, vixen power. Every guy fantasizes about being with one, and a good share of women fantasize about being one. So make tonight the night. Make a dinner date together and rent your favorite James Bond film. When it's over, she becomes the Bond Girl, slipping into something ultrasexy and luring him into her sexy web of intrigue and adventure.

TURNING TRICKS

Here's an oldie but goodie: On a night when the kids are sleeping out somewhere else, she dresses up like a street hooker, fishnets and all, and sneaks out the back door. She then rings the doorbell, and when he answers, she tells him she's been sent here to make his every fantasy come true—even giving a price list for her special services and talking as dirty as she can without cracking each of them up too much.

NURSE BETTY

There isn't a man on the planet who doesn't like to be babied—and who better to baby them than a sexy nurse? Devise a nurse costume, complete with cap and thigh-high white stockings with a short little white uniform. You can even check out your local costume retailer or even a lingerie store, like Fredericks of Hollywood, which features fetishy-type ensembles like these. When fully decked out, she takes his temperature and reports that he is, indeed, quite ill. And then she nurses him back to health with passion, taking control of the entire sexy situation.

FOXY LADY

"Foxy Lady" by Jimi Hendrix is a fun song to act out during sexplay. She can pretend she's a 1960s hippie, swept up in the fury of the sexual revolution and ready to push the boundaries of the establishment right into the next decade. Or play it more conservatively, just dancing around seductively when the song plays. It's entirely up to you and your comfort level. Just put on the song and see where the music takes you.

Just for Her . . .

Do blondes have more fun? It's time to find out. Go to your local wig shop and buy yourself a blond wig. If you're already a blonde, make it a platinum blond wig and stash it away till morning. When you wake, head to the bathroom, throw it on, and secure it well. Now get yourself into character. Fantasize that you are Marilyn Monroe, Pamela Anderson . . . whoever makes you feel the most empowered and the sexiest. Pretend that he's a big-shot movie producer and you're a starlet desperate to be cast in his next film. Now jump on top of him and show him just how badly you want it.

BORN-AGAIN VIRGIN

She's a schoolgirl, complete with hair in pigtails, short pleated skirt, white blouse—buttoned one button short of purely innocent—knee socks, and white cotton panties. She takes him off guard, perhaps telling him to come for lunch one day and surprising him in this outfit. She innocently tells him she's a virgin and wants him to be her first. When he takes her, she stays in character, continuing to act innocent and maybe even a little shocked. Until he awakens in her everything she hoped this could be.

WHITE NIGHT

In a variation of the above, the woman pretends it's her wedding night. She wears all white—something lacy, demure, and virginal—and makes sure he gets a good look at her in her pristine white lingerie before climbing into bed next to him and turning out the light. Like the schoolgirl, she really hams it up, pretending she's nervous and so happy to be giving it up to him, and he acts wordly and protective and suave as he takes her. She can play that she's really scared and wants to stop; he can insist that she's his property now and he's going to take what's rightfully his. . . . Which actually starts to move us out of the realm of role-play and into the world of playful bondage, where boundaries are pushed all the time to the delight of each partner. But we'll get more into this in the next chapter.

Like a Virgin

If you really want to go "virginal," there are some products available designed to make the vagina seem tighter.

- **Vaginal cones** are small, tamponlike weights designed to be slipped into the vagina and used when a woman is going about her daily activities, for fifteen minutes twice a day. She inserts the cone and squeezes her vagina muscles to hold the device in place. The idea is to start with the lightest cone, and once she can hold that without too much squeezing, she moves on to the next size until she gets to the heaviest one. And by that time, she'll be so tight it will be like prom night all over again.
- **Neuromuscular electrical stimulation (NMES)** is a special procedure in which a probe is inserted into the vagina to stimulate the muscles of the pelvic floor with an electric current, which causes them to tighten and loosen. The treatments are done either at your doctor's office or on a home device and happen for twenty minutes every one to four days for a number of weeks.
- **Neocontrol** is done in a chair that stimulates the muscles of the pelvic floor using magnetic fields for twenty to thirty minutes at a time, at your doctor's office, a couple of times a week for a couple of months.
- **Shrink cream** doesn't hurt, but it also doesn't work all that well. It enhances the sensation, making your vagina feel more sensitive, but I don't think it actually shrinks anything. Still, if you're not interested in cones or treatments, it may be an option for you. It may not be for everyone, however, as it's made from chemicals. Those who prefer a more "natural" method of tightening should stick with the Kegels.

THE NASTY NANNY

Just because she's female doesn't mean she has to be submissive! There are lots of fun ways for the woman to control the action—like this scenario. The guy's wife is away for the weekend (or maybe she left him or died—all that matters is that she's not in the picture) and he's hired a stern, pinched shrew of a woman who wears shapeless drab clothing, her hair pulled tightly into a bun that she pins low to cover the back of her neck, to take care of his unruly children.

But appearances are deceiving, which he learns one night after the kids are fast asleep. She enters the living room, where he's made a mess—beer cans, potato chips, whatever—and sternly chides him for his sloppiness. She orders him to clean up. She slaps him on the tush if he's at all insolent. Once he's picked things up nearly to her satisfaction, she bends over in front of him to show him some mess he missed, revealing under her frumpy shirt not a stitch of underwear. Knowing she's got his attention, she strips off her clothes and takes down her hair, revealing a goddess in disguise. He stops to admire her, and she admonishes him, telling him he is now punished and will have to do whatever she asks to get back into her good graces. Whatever she wants is what she requests—and he has no choice but to deliver. Or else!

PRIVATE DANCER

In a strip club, a patron can get a private lap dance by one of the strippers for about twenty bucks. Sometimes there's even contact involved, which is usually her gyrating and pulsating all over him—but he's not allowed to touch. At home, she can give a lap dance that can blow any of the pros away, because

The Forbidden Dance

Dancing is great foreplay—for her and him—so why not indulge. If going out dancing is out of character for you, all the better reason to put on your dancing shoes and investigate the options. You may discover new sides to yourselves that will make you giggle and only bring you closer.

When you hit the dance floor, dance as close and sexually with each other as possible—really push the limits of your public comfort level. After a sweaty, sexy night like this, you'll be revved up and ready to finish off with some extra-special sexplay.

not only does she know exactly how to touch and caress and squeeze him until he explodes— but he can touch her, too. All it takes is a little sexy music and a lot of imagination. And even a twenty-dollar bill stuffed in her panties or bra (if she's even wearing one) if you want to make it really authentic.

HEAD CHEERLEADER

He's the star quarterback in a horrible career slump. She's the head cheerleader whose raison d'être is the happiness and success of the team—and to do whatever it takes to get the players up to speed and performing at their peak. And now it's his turn to get a dose of her brand of spirit—and maybe get his own "spirit stick" off while he's at it. . . .

She comes into the locker room, where he's sitting alone in a towel. She's all decked out in her uniform, pom-poms and all. She approaches him and starts swinging her pom-poms, cheering, and jumping up and down. Which is when he realizes she isn't wearing anything under that uniform.

"What do you want?" she cheers. "What do you need?" she commands. And his towel somehow mysteriously falls to the floor. As she bends over to pick it up, he guides her head to his exposed member and tells her to go to town, and she eagerly, hungrily complies. And as she bends over his lap, taking him all in, he reaches under her skirt, penetrating her with one, two, three fingers, fondling her furiously as she goes down on him. And before they know it, each experiences the touchdown of their lives!

SHE-BOSS

She's a high-powered executive, he's the mailroom clerk who lost a very important package that she needs replaced, so she calls him to her office immediately. She sits in her executive chair with her feet sexily perched on the desk, her ankles crossed on one impossibly high-heeled pump dangling from the toes of her top foot. She makes him stand in front of her desk as she chides and scolds him, diminishing him with her words as she dominates him with her eyes and her mind.

She tells him how important that package was to her and demands he whip out his own package out to see if it will make a suitable replacement. He obliges and stands naked from the waist down before her. She slinks from behind her desk and inspects the package, first with her hand and then with her mouth. Getting him almost to the brink of orgasm as she samples his stick, she pulls away and tells him this is not a sufficient test. She then kneels on her desk, keeping on her impossibly high heels, and demands that he push his package right into her so she can confirm with absolute certainty that this package of his will indeed do.

DO YOU TAKE *DICK*-TATION?

Most of the fantasies we've charted out so far are from her point of view—but what about him? Here's a sexy scenario in which he gets to call the shots as the big boss and she must do what he says—everything he says—or risk losing her job.

As a high-powered executive, he is probably wearing a suit. But as a lowly assistant, she wears what she can afford—a too-short skirt and no undies, which simply cost too much. He's called her in for a meeting to discuss her insolence at asking for a raise, and to reprimand her for turning on everyone in the office every time she bends over her cabinet to file paperwork.

What you do from here is your own fantasy. Does she need to be spanked over his knee? Does he need to give her a special kind of lashing—a tongue-lashing—to instruct her in the ways of proper office etiquette? See where your imagination takes you.

PIZZA'S HERE!

This scenario can work with the man dominating or being dominated. And he doesn't have to be a pizza delivery guy. He could be a plumber coming to service her pipes or an electrician coming to charge up her voltage. Whatever you decide, just have fun!

If he's a pizza boy who's late on his delivery, she can refuse to tip him. Unless he shows her another way he can earn it. If he's a plumber, maybe he has a pipe he needs her to hold on to while he works. An electrician could have been called to service her vibrator, which she just can't seem to get to work right. . . .

Whatever the scenario, she should answer the door in a towel or skimpy robe—in either case, wearing nothing underneath. If he's in trouble, she barks orders at him until he acceptably does what she wants.

On the male-dominating side, she could be getting in his way. Maybe she talks too much and needs her piehole plugged up with his special pipe, or wire, or pepperoni. Whatever the case, he's going to show her that even though she's paying him for his services, he—and only he—calls the shots.

THE POSTMAN ALWAYS RINGS TWICE

He rings the doorbell, and when she answers, he tells her he has a special package she must sign for, but she must open the door immediately, as he cannot simply leave it for her and only her signature will be accepted. When she lets him in, he whips out his "package" and takes her right there—on the kitchen countertop, hall table, you name it.

SLAVE 4 U

Tomorrow morning, as you're racing off to work, hand your partner a special note that reads "Slave 4 U"—like the Britney Spears song. Then lean in and whisper in their ear that they are to meet you in the bedroom tonight at ten o'clock sharp, and that this is the last demand you will be able to make of them until six o'clock the following morning. Tell them to spend the day thinking of all the ways you can please them later—and to not work late tonight.

During the game, if your partner suggests something you aren't comfortable with, tell them, but see how far you are willing to push your comfort level in the name of their pleasure. You may surprise yourself with what you're capable of when you choose to relax, trust, and just enjoy.

THE SWASHBUCKLER

Pirates are the gypsies of the seas and they are known for taking what they want. And what woman doesn't like to be taken? So go to your local costume shop or buy your costume online, and surprise her the next chance you get with your pirate hat and sword. Tell her she now belongs to you and is your prisoner. You will protect her from the rest of the crew, but there is a price for that protection. The price is sex . . . sex all day with you.

THE POOL BOY

Pool or no pool, you can do this, guys. All you have to do is put on your swimsuit, a tank top, and some dark shades. Perhaps slather yourself with suntan lotion for a sexy scent and to make your skin all soft and slippery.

In the middle of the afternoon, maybe on a weekend, ring the doorbell with a towel in hand. Let your lady know that you're here to clean the pool. If you don't have a pool, insist that you do and just pretend it's there. Pool or none, start cleaning, and when you get really hot and sweaty, take off your clothes. Now call her outside and tell her there's a problem with the pool light . . . a big one. Take her right there on the grass or in the water.

WOMANIZER, WOMANIZER, WOMANIZER...

Like the Britney Spears song, every woman fantasizes about being with a man who's smooth and got the moves. And how does one get "the moves"? Well, any guy who's got them has probably been around the block more than a few times, and he has probably talked a lot of women out of their panties before they even knew what was happening to them.

So, guys, you're going to have to make this believable and dress the part, à la James Bond. Seriously, don a tuxedo and show her your smoothest moves and pull out all your sexiest one-liners. Have her meet you at a bar and pick your lady up. Take her home and make love to her the way you think James would. Hint: Nice and slow and adoring of every part of her.

THE MILE-HIGH CLUB

Does anyone really have sex in airplanes? That's for you to find out—if you dare. But for the purposes of this chapter, it's all about make-believe. And it's all going to take place right in your own home. Here are a few scenarios to enact:

Moon over Miami

You're honeymooners fresh from your wedding reception and heading to some sunny island, where you plan to celebrate your marriage by walking around half-naked, sipping tropical cocktails, and consummating your union. Over and over and over again. Trouble is, the flight is six hours long and you sit there adoring your partner across your pretend airline seat, which, for your purposes, can be the living room couch, and you know there's no way you can wait. . . . So you don't.

At first you try and keep your lust discreet at your seat, fondling each other under the blankets that are sometimes handed out, or the small flight pillows as you futilely try and balance them on your laps. Then one of you excuses yourself to go to the restroom and tells the other to wait sixty seconds—and then to join you.

Do you have a small guest powder room? That's the bathroom you want to use, and the smaller the better. Just like in an airplane bathroom, you will need to be standing—and things will need to happen quickly. Whether this means both partners are standing, her back resting up against the wall for leverage, her sitting on the edge of the sink and him standing before her, or her bent over the sink with her skirt or dress tossed up and over her lower back—well, that's entirely up to you!

Strangers in the Night

You and your partner are business travelers who have to take intercontinental flights almost weekly. You've been doing this for so long, you move yourself along on automatic pilot, barely noticing anything about your trip. Except for the sexy stranger you see each and every week at the cocktail lounge before takeoff; on the endless security line; across the aisle and up a few rows from you in business class. You've never spoken a word to each other, but from the looks you exchange, you both know what you want.

One of you will walk by the other on your way to the restroom, but you still will not speak. All you will do is nod your head, raise your eyebrows, or even gesture in the direction of the restroom. You will enter and wait. And when your sexy stranger joins you, there's still no talking.

Whatever positions worked while you were honeymooners will work now, but because you are strangers, there is no love here, only white-hot, savage lust. You are free to be as greedy to satisfy your own needs as you please. You don't want to know anything about the other. You just want to savor and enjoy these few lusty moments you experience as you tear away at each other with a passion you've never experienced before, and never will again. . . . Until you fly next week, that is.

So That's Why They Call It a Cockpit!

Now you're not lovers and you're not strangers—you're colleagues. One of you is a pilot and one of you is a flight attendant, but it doesn't matter which. (Perhaps the one who feels like being the dominant partner can be the pilot this time, and you can switch off later if you like this game.) Let's make him the pilot this time.

You've been working this same flight together for years. You've always been attracted to each other, but the airline has a policy against staff being in relationships, so you've never been able to act on it. The sweet, sexy tension has been mounting for some time now, and you're both about to explode.

So when she enters the cockpit this time, and he's somehow, for the first time, completely alone, and she's forgotten to button up her blouse all the way—exposing the lacey edge of a red satin bra—he can contain himself no longer. He sets the plane to fly on automatic pilot and takes her, right there on the console. Whether in missionary or doggie style is up to them. He takes her hard, like he's never taken any woman before, and they soon are moaning and screaming in ecstasy. But wait—did he accidentally flip the PA switch, so that everything they've been doing has now been broadcast to the entire flight? As they collapse in a sweaty, sated heat, they just don't seem to care at all. . . . Whatever the consequences, it was worth it!

MY HERO!

She is a damsel in distress. Perhaps she's trapped in a burning building or tied to the railroad tracks by some dastardly villain and the four-forty-five is about to come through. Perhaps it's as simple as her kitty Friskers being trapped up in a tree and needing some strong, brave man to rescue it. Whatever the reason, she's in trouble and needs to be saved. And he, the dashing hero—in a fireman's or policeman's uniform, or just some guy off the street—he's going to swoop in and do whatever it takes to save her. Somehow she is very poor. Her wallet burned in the building, the villain robbed her, her cat used her money as litter, causing her to chase the thing up the tree in the first place—whatever the case, she has nothing to reward him with except her undying gratitude. . . . And how that will manifest itself sexually is entirely up to him.

MONSTER MASH

One of the things that is so exciting about the vampire romances so popular these days is the idea of being taken by a force that is otherwordly—as dark as it is dangerous, and completely dominating. No mortal woman can resist the charms of a dashing demon, even if entangling herself in his web could mean certain death or eternal damnation.

He can be a vampire, but it doesn't really matter. Something with high levels of animal magnetism, like a shapeshifter or werewolf, would also do (though a zombie or mummy may not be too sexy). She is as innocent as a spring lamb, fast asleep in her white nightgown as she dreams of butterflies and flowers. He, in costume (or at least in fangs and cape, which can easily and innocently be purchased at your local party-supply or costume store), storms into her room like he owns the place and sees her fast asleep. And he must, MUST have her.

With terrifying speed (it's possible he even flew), he pounces on the bed and onto his prey, tearing her nightgown off and ripping her panties at the seams. "No, no!" she half-cries as she opens her mouth and her legs to accept him—his otherwordly, larger-than-life, paranormally huge package. And all the while as he takes her, without mercy, she begs him to stop. And to continue. And to stop. Until the climax of her life washes over her and she becomes forever his.

NOW YOU KNOW...

Fantasy and role-play can really cement a relationship as they push you past what you think are your limits of trust and fun and therefore bring you closer together. And now, speaking of pressing past limits, get ready to have some fun with light, playful bondage in the next chapter. Unrestrained pleasures derived through, well, using restraints. Talk about kinky.

Kinkiest

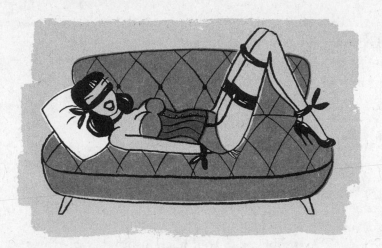

Chapter 9

Tie Me Up, Tie You Up

Now we head into the kinkiest of the kinky that two people can do to one another, and still face each other the next morning. . . .

In all seriousness, the activities in this chapter—and the rest of this section—are not for everyone. If the suggestions here don't appeal to you, it doesn't mean you haven't been kinky enough. All it means is that you and your partner have found your high-water mark and are happy with your limits. And that's absolutely fine.

But for the rest of you . . .

Traditionally, SM is a power play of dominant over submissive; of a "sadist" controlling the actions, but much to the "masochist's" delight. And that's the most important thing to remember. When you experiment with bondage, both partners, in whatever role, must ultimately feel *delight*. If there's anything else going on—coercion, fear, dread, anxiety—this kind of play must end right away.

All that being said, you need several things in place to engage in and enjoy the offerings presented in this chapter. The first, as we touched on above, is the unconditional consent of both partners. Once you have that, the right attitude is key. Bondage is supposed to be fun and sexually enhancing. If it is in any way frightening or unpleasantly uncomfortable, it's not working. If both partners are not having a good time or if one partner is doing something that truly hurts the other partner mentally or physically, it's going to create more problems in your relationship than anything else. But when all factors align, it can be a delightful method to play out and enjoy some of your wildest fantasies.

Look back at the last chapter. Perhaps you'd like the idea of being ravaged by a pirate or dominated by a woman in power. Whatever the case may be, don't just wing it. Talk about what gets you hot before you embark, about what titillates and what terrifies, and then let go and enjoy this very intimate way to get to know and enjoy your lover in a whole new way.

> ## Naughty Nibble
>
> Be sure to have a safe word that both of you know and understand—something one of you says aloud when it's time for your partner to stop doing whatever it is they are doing. I have friends who use the word "pineapple," but you choose something that works for you. Just not "stop" or "no," as these kind of defeat the purpose: Screaming out "no" is part of the game; it doesn't mean to stop—in fact, it only fuels the action.

ANIMAL MAGNETISM

Let's put a new spin on role-playing. This time, you're going to pretend like you're an animal. Not just any old animal, but one of the sexiest, slinkiest animals imaginable—a cat. You can buy a bondage collar to wear around your neck, though a large-size cat or dog collar that you can easily pick up in your local grocery or pet store can also do the trick. Just place it around your neck and start to purr and slink around, rubbing up against your "person" and letting them know that they totally *own* you. Me-ow. And what they do to you or what they make you do is up to the two of you. Your partner could insist you wear a leash. Maybe they'd like to see you lap up a bowl of milk on the floor with you on all fours. Is it time to "crate" the naughty dog or kitty? Seriously—it's up to you.

SEE NO EVIL

One of the best ways to heighten the senses is to take a sense away, which is why a blindfold is such a kinky sex prop. Take away your lover's sight and the rest of her senses work harder, making the experience that much more intense.

There are many options in blindfolds available—even fabricated in red and black leather and decorated with spikes and other crazy embellishments (more for you than the blindfoldee)—but a silk or satin scarf you already have in the closet makes a pretty good blindfold as well. Let your lover choose the blindfold they want to wear and have them put it on. But your lover's control of the situation ends there.

Carefully guide your lover around while he or she is wearing the blindfold and don't let them crash. This is how you build trust. Lead them to a quiet room, where their trust will now pay off. Take off the blindfold to allow your lover to see every lusciously decadent thing you will be doing to them—or leave it on to keep the sexy mystery alive. It's whatever works for you guys.

HOT 'N' COLD

You're going to need a blindfold, a bowl of ice cubes, and a couple of lit candlesticks for this scenario. First, blindfold your lover and then guide them to the bed, where they are to lie down. Now strip off each article of clothing, slowly and seductively, piece by piece. Or, if you want to create more urgency, tear away at your lover's garments, really putting them in the frame of mind that they are at your mercy.

Now stand above your lover and, taking an ice cube in your hand, let ice-cold droplets tickle his or her body from about two feet above. Now take the candle and let hot wax fall in different areas from where the water dripped. Just be sure to hold the candle at least four feet above, to give the wax enough time to cool from scalding to just plain warm when it hits your lover's skin. (In fact, you may want to test the distance on yourself first.) It's important that the drops hit in different places, as not knowing where the next drop falls will only heighten your partner's senses and make the seduction that much sweeter.

Naughty Nibble

If you are using handcuffs, make sure that they don't actually *require* keys to open—that if keys are involved at all, they are simply part of the "game." You don't want to end up in the position of having to explain to a locksmith what happened when you lose the keys and can't get the cuffs open.

CAN'T CUFF ENOUGH

Furry handcuffs. Leather handcuffs. Wrist cuffs made with Velcro fasteners. Even a plain old pair of panty hose. They can all make for some great wrist restraints. If you've never tied your partner up before, start slowly, loosely tying their wrists together, then working up to tying them more securely—and to other things. Just make sure your partner is into it before you secure even the first knot. Talk about what's going to happen and be sure they aren't scared or feeling compromised in any way. And then have a good time with it.

TAKE NO PRISONERS—OR MAYBE JUST THE ONE . . .

Check out sex-toy catalogs for wrist-to-waist cuffs. These keep your partner's hands loosely attached to his waist—like he's a prisoner in a chain gang. They can't really move their arms, so you can control whether they touch you or not. But your lover will still have some freedom of movement, which may make them more comfortable about things. Now lead your lover around and decide what you'd like for them to do to earn your merciful pardon. As a side note: Be sure to buy the wrist-to-waist cuffs with the Velcro ties, as they are fairly easy to get out of. Remember—we're dealing with the illusion of being a prisoner here, not the real thing.

ALL TIED UP

Ladies—he'll be bound to love you after you try this trick on him. With some neckties or scarves, tie your lover to a chair. Now put on a show that will drive him crazy and make him lust for you forever.

Undress as sexily as possible in front of him only to expose the hot lacy bra and

> ### Naughty Nibble
> When tying up your lover, never bind the restraints too tightly and always bind in positions your partner can move around in. To get the most out of bondage play, take it slowly and remember you don't have to be uncomfortable to enjoy yourselves. It's much more important that you are both comfy and happy.

Just for Her . . .

Here are the top strip performances in film you can emulate as you gyrate for your guy:

Jamie Lee Curtis in *True Lies*
Kim Basinger in *9¹/₂ Weeks*
Salma Hayek in *From Dusk Till Dawn*
Elisha Cuthbert in *The Girl Next Door*
Natalie Portman in *Closer*

---

panties you have underneath, then prance around the room for a while before you take them off. Sit on top of him and pleasure yourself so he can get a great view but can't touch. He is tied up, after all. Now turn around and give him a backside view. Take a break to apply your favorite sweet-smelling massage oil all over your body, massage your breasts and run them over his chest and lower extremities, oil up your tush and straddle him. Gyrate over his privates with your tush facing him. All this gyrating will probably have made you pretty hot by now, so why not place him inside you and ride, baby ride.

NO TOUCHING, PLEASE

Tie his wrists only to the bedposts. Do you realize how hard it is for him to not be able to use his hands? If you don't have bedposts, tie his hands together and have him lie on his tummy. Mount him like you're riding a horse and pretend to be doing just that. Rock back and forth, whispering sweet naughty things in his ears and tickling the sides of his torso until he just can't stand it any longer. Now allow him to turn over. For the grand finale, I want you to kiss every square inch of the front of his body—saving the best for last.

CAPTIVE AUDIENCE

Tie your lover to a chair. Now get out your favorite spanking tool—a wooden spoon, a hairbrush, or a paddle you picked up at a sex shop—and start disciplining. Think of five ridiculous or even funny things you can reprimand your partner about. Perhaps he's in trouble for forgetting to put the toilet seat down, or maybe she forgot to undress in front of you last night—very naughty indeed. Every time you bring to light one of your partner's faux pas, give him or her a tiny little spank on the knee, shoulder, or top of the thigh. *Remember when you left the dishes in the sink? Bad girl.* <spank>. *Remember when you looked at that woman with lustful eyes? Such a naughty boy.* <spank>. Enjoy coming up with your own personal ones. Remember, this is supposed to be ridiculous.

For the climax, insist your partner tell you how sorry they are. Untie them and tell them they will need to earn your forgiveness—and then tell them how. If you're feeling particularly dominating, leave them tied up and let them know the only way they're going to learn is through the proper punishment—and leave them tied as you drill this lesson in.

THE BUTLER DID ME

Guys—get your woman off in two ways. One, by getting some housework done. The other, by making it impossible to lift a finger to help . . . you or herself.

Tie her ankles and wrists with soft scarves or bandannas and have her sit on the couch, naked, while you do some arbitrary housework naked. Dust off the table in front of her. Vacuum the room—whatever comes to mind. After about ten or so minutes, tell her you'd like her to kneel, facing the couch, or to bend over one of the sides. With a clean, or better yet, new duster, the kind with feathers, dust her neck and back and bottom and legs and tickle her with it. Heighten her senses and really make her nuts. And now that she thinks you're totally nuts . . . take her from behind as slowly and sensuously as possible.

Naughty Nibble

Bondage tape is not only really easy to use, it also comes off easily and quickly. You can use it to tie up your lover's wrists and ankles—or her wrists to her ankles. She can bind her breasts, he can bind his package (the visual turns some people on)—and you can even use it as a gag if you feel that adventurous. Just take out a spool and see where your imaginations lead.

DOM SEXY!

In this scenario, she must wear a latex outfit—which is exactly what a dominatrix would wear and exactly what she is right now. Nearby, she should have a paddle and a rubber whip. And now the real fun begins: She tells him to take off all his clothes, and he must obey, immediately, or suffer the consequences. She then instructs him to kneel before her and, with paddle in hand, tell him he's been very, very bad. She gently spanks him on the bottom with her paddle, and if she does not feel that's been punishment enough, she reaches for the whip and says that it's high time she whipped him into shape. (Just be sure never to hit your lover in the face or in the genital area—just the butt, arms, legs, and back.)

NOW YOU KNOW . . .

Can you reward and punish your lover at the same time? Of course you can—and have a great time doing it. The most important things are to always be aware of how your actions are affecting your partner, and to not drink heavily or do drugs if you're involved in any kind of bondage play. You need to keep all your senses sharp, which will make the experience that much more pleasurable anyway. Especially if you're thinking of filming things . . . but that's the next chapter.

naughty nibble

Corsets are very common with this type of play. Latex and corsets really help set the mood and take you out of yourself and into the fantasy.

Chapter 10

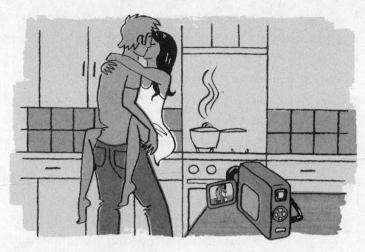

Lights, Camera, and a Whole Lot of Action

n this chapter, we'll be exploring tons of ways to be kinky that would not have been possible even twenty years ago. Thanks to so many fabulous advances in technology, there are countless options available now for us to explore uncharted erotic realms, and in the privacy of our own homes, like watching—and even *creating*—adult films.

Does porn freak you out? Some of it should, sure, but there's also a plethora of it that isn't so scary. There are "how to," instructional sex videos and soft-core films, which show little, leaving more to the imagination. And then there's hard-core, which puts it all out there. Some porn tells a story, while some has no point except to deliver cheap, shocking thrills— which is not necessarily a bad thing. There's man-on-woman, woman-on-woman, group . . . You get it. Everything you can think of, someone has made it. Oh, did I mention there are even porn cartoons?

So how do you know what's going to be right for you? Research. If you're overwhelmed by all the choices available, start out by tracking down a book called *The Ultimate Guide to Adult Videos*. It's a handy resource that tells you everything you ever wanted to know about any porn movie out there.

How you get your adult films really depends on your comfort level. If you have cable TV or satellite, you can order movies via your remote control and never have to speak to another human being about it. Hit the Internet to privately investigate all the options, and even download from various erotic websites. And if you're feeling particularly brave, visit a love boutique or adult video store. Just keep in mind that while love boutiques tend to be more women-friendly, they don't always have much to offer in terms of porn aside from perhaps a step up from what Hollywood will give you. On the other hand, an adult video store has just about everything, and if you're not too embarrassed to ask, there's usually a knowledgeable clerk eager to break it down for you.

As you explore this brave new world with your lover, please keep in mind that porn is not meant to replace "the real thing"; it's an enhancement. If you feel like you're starting to fixate on porn and would rather spend time with your remote control or computer mouse than your

Naughty Nibble

On your next "date night," visit an adult novelty store with your partner. Each of you should pick out things you think the other should have. Lace or latex underwear, a new sex toy, a steamy DVD, some flavored lube, a pair of clear heels . . . Just have a good time with it.

partner, it's time to cease and desist. Porn is for foreplay. It's an "igniter" and a resource for ideas and new things to try. It can even help you out when you might not be totally "in the mood" and want to get there quickly.

Now, while the title of this chapter suggests it may be all about adult videos, it isn't just about porn. It's also about erotic readings, taking photos, exploring the Wild Wicked Web, and just having a good time. Because there are plenty of laughs just waiting to be had while you investigate all the offerings in this tawdry world, it's sure to keep the love in your relationship, um, well-lubed.

CHEAP SHOTS

Here's an activity that isn't quite so innocent. . . . One day make it a point to snap photos of each other just looking hot. By this I mean more than sitting pretty. I mean looking sexy—doing sexy things, like her lapping away at a melting ice cream cone, him lasciviously licking the inside of a peach. Of course, they don't have to be too overtly sexual. For example, make him dinner with a much-too-mini skirt on, or in your underwear or slightly open robe (exposing that there's nothing being worn underneath), or even in a button-up shirt that's barely buttoned.

Take the photos and make an album of them, and look at the album together as you share your thoughts and fantasies. "I like how you're circling the tip of that cucumber—do you think you could . . ." et cetera. By all means add to it as often as you want; just be sure you go through it at least once a month. These types of exchanges boost self-esteem and in turn your sex life—not to mention that it makes for some fun, subtle foreplay.

INSTANT GRATIFICATION

Not everyone has a Polaroid camera anymore, but most people have the next-best thing when it comes to "instant photo gratification": a digital camera. Knowing that you can take photos of anything you want, and that these photos will not be processed by some technician in a photo-developing lab somewhere, really helps knock those pesky inhibitions away.

So how will you embrace this opportunity? Will you play male photographer and lingerie model? Female photographer and wild man found in the jungle? Or just play it straight, each of you taking sexy photos of each other in various stages of undress? Whatever you decide, just enjoy yourself and be free about it. After your session, review the shots and delete or discard as many as you want. The ones you save can be stashed away in a safe place to savor and enjoy at another time—either as just a little treat of eye candy or as an invitation to a tryst. You decide.

Naughty Nibble

Take advantage of every opportunity technology has to offer. Use your cell phone to take a sexy photo of yourself and text it to your love. And if you have a really advanced phone, create a teasing video clip. What dirty message can you convey in fifteen, thirty, or sixty seconds?

SECRET ALBUM

Create an all-nude album featuring photos of yourself and your partner that you store in your bedroom under lock and key. The naked part is mandatory: Just how graphically naked you decide to make it is between you and your partner. Take pictures of each other tied up in colorful latex tape. Paint each other all over with acrylic body paints. Focus on "favorite body parts." Dedicate the album exclusively to his penis or her breasts. Again, it's entirely up to you.

CARNAL COLLAGE

Several years ago, my boyfriend—now husband—was going to be away for a span of time and begged me to send him erotic photos of myself via the Internet. I decided to create an erotic collage of photos, some naked and some not, and e-mailed it to him. Needless to say, the concept of "out of sight, out of mind" went right out the window.

Why not give this a try yourself? You can include as many photos as you like or a few. Keep in mind that you want there to be enough so that your partner has a satisfying selection to savor, but not so many that the pictures are so small they can't see any of the good stuff.

THROUGH HER EYES

These days, the porn industry is no longer a male-dominated world. Plenty of female directors have thrown their hat in the ring and come up with some excellent erotic offerings. For example, Candida Royalle directs porn that is great for first-time viewers. Her stuff is well-filmed, has a story, and includes both romance and somewhat explicit sex scenes—but not hard-core explicit. It's essentially porn from a woman's perspective. Check it out, but don't forget to take it all lightly. Remember: This is more about fun than it is about the sex.

ARE YOU GAME?

One of the least-intimidating and most exciting ways to bring adult films into your relationship is to make a game of it—really capitalize on sharing the experience together. Here are some ideas:

Porn for Women

Dinner Party, directed by Cameron Grant

Velvet Tension, Velvet Thrust, Ranch House Lust, produced by InPulse Productions

Chemistry Series, Vols. 1–3, directed by Tristan Taormino

The Eyes of Desire Series, 1 and 2, by Candida Royalle

The Bridal Shower, by Candida Royalle

Afrodite Superstar, by Candida Royalle

- Every time someone in the movie sighs and says "Oh God," beat your partner to the punch—with a light punch on the arm. Whoever throws the first punch earns one sexy kiss wherever they want, right then and there. Tally up the punches at the end of the film, and whoever's thrown the most gets to enjoy a long, luscious sexual favor at the expense of the loser. But truly, are there any losers here?
- As you watch an adult movie together, make some notes, focusing on some of your favorite parts. When the movie ends, exchange your notes, see if there are any activities you can agree to try together, and get down to it.
- During the movie, press pause every time you see something you like and talk about why. Either show your partner why right there and then, or prolong the ecstasy until after the movie—whatever the situation calls for.

- Tie your lover to a chair and "force" him or her to watch *their* favorite porn scene—as you do your best to simulate it in the flesh.

SEX ED 101

If porn seems too raw for you, try renting a sexy sex-education video. Instructional videos are some of the best tools for experiencing sex on film without having to actually order or purchase the rough stuff. And you can have lots of fun with it. If you ever wanted to know more about the G-spot, here's a semirespectable way to find out, right? It's "for educational purposes," after all.

Porn for Men

Deep Throat, Gerard Rocco Damiano

Young Sluts #20, Hustler

Farmer's Filthy Li'l Daughter #2, Hustler

Anal Perversions, Hustler

Cookies & Milf #3, Hustler

Hustler's Lesbian Fantasies, Hustler

There's a lot more out there for men than women. It really all depends on his tastes. Other DVDs he may like include *The Green Door* with the late Marilyn Chambers and *The Devil in Miss Jones*, also directed by Gerard Damiano. There's also the *Girls Gone Wild* series, which isn't all hard-core porn but still gets the guys going. (Just don't use your credit card to pay for this one.)

Just for Her . . .

Tell your guy it's time to go shopping and don't tell him where. Then surprise him by taking him to the nearest sex shop. Pick out a porno together—even several—and head home quickly to watch them. It may not be your cup of tea, what with all that raw, graphic action and bad lighting and music, but we're not expecting Oscar contenders here. The point is to watch them with him, who more often than not really enjoys them, and pick out an act or position you'd both like to try. And I guarantee there will be something. Ahh, the power of porn.

Here's a great way to get off on sex ed. The minute you get turned on watching the film, pause it and start fooling around. As soon as you are about to orgasm, stop what you're doing and resume watching the video. Allow your excitement to simmer down and then heat up again for about five minutes or so. Then pause the video and get back into it—

Just for Him . . .

If, when watching a dirty movie, your lover continues to make comments like "That's disgusting" or "I can't believe I'm watching this," it's possible you've chosen something a bit too hard-core for her. Change the video, or, even better, take the opportunity to talk to her about it and find out why. If she hasn't demanded you turn off the movie or left the room in disgust, there's a chance she's intrigued by what she's watching; she's just a little shocked and trying to process it all. Remember: She's just not as "visual" as you are.

but before you climax, stop what you're doing and turn the video back on. While this might seem terribly annoying on paper, what you're doing in actuality is intensifying your ultimate climax by stalling it.

AS SEEN ON TV

Tonight, rent a porno and watch it under the sheets with your partner, holding hands—and that's it—the entire time. Every time something turns you on, give your partner's hand a light little squeeze and have him or her do the same to you. If your partner never squeezes, it might be time to try a different film, which is why it's useful to have more than one on hand: Perhaps one educational, one soft-core, and one that's beyond naughty. Hey, you never know.

Motel Sex

Book a night at a cheap motel and ask your lover to rendezvous with you there after work. Tell them there's something there you absolutely must show them—and that it's a surprise. And don't forget to give them the room number.

Plan to arrive at least fifteen minutes before your partner, and take this opportunity to put on the absolutely tackiest sex "outfit" you can find—comically slutty lingerie for her, or, for him, perhaps a pair of leopard-print briefs that hug him in just the right places. Now get into bed with a chilled six-pack of beer (cans, naturally). The minute your partner opens the door, yell: Surprise. Now suggest he or she hop into bed with you, select a porno to watch together, and make hot nasty motel sex with the movie playing in the background.

A WHOLE NEW LEVEL

What if regular movies or TV actually let you see what happened to characters when everything fades to black during a love scene? Why not make it up yourselves? Reenact love scenes from your favorite TV shows or movies, and make the super-porn version. Show 'em how it's really done. Imagine how they did it and then just do it. And don't forget to videotape the scenes for future bonding.

A CLICK AWAY . . .

Instead of watching TV tonight, suggest to your partner that you surf the Internet together to do some "essential research." There are thousands of sex-education sites designed to teach couples how to make more satisfying love, including www.drnatasha.com. Tell your partner you're interested in

Cyber HotSpots

Check out the following websites with your partner tonight. You're guaranteed to find a new experience, something neither of you has ever done before but will be desperate to try:

- tablesexwithsue.com
- drruth.com
- the-clitoris.com
- the-penis.com
- hustler.com
- playboy.com
- masturbationpage.com
- playcouples.com

brushing up on what you know to become a better lover. Now explore, explore, explore, asking your partner to point out techniques and positions he or she finds intriguing. Once you've had enough learning, head to bed and put those lessons into practice.

CHAT ROOM

With today's technology and a little anonymity, you and your lover can enjoy checking out sexy chat rooms together to explore what other couples are doing and maybe to learn something new. And who knows—all you may end up taking away from the experience is sharing a lot of laughs, and there's no harm in that.

GIRLS—AND GUYS—ON FILM

Set up your video camera, not to tape, just to view yourselves on your TV screen. Point it toward your bed and start going at it, watching yourselves on screen as you make hot, passionate nooky. Experiment with different positions, ones that give you good angles and views.

> ## naughty nibble
> Everyone knows the game Guitar Hero. What if you played it naked—and filmed each other while you were at it? Ahhh, the memories.

NOW, THAT'S A FILM *STRIP*

Much of the time, stripteases are the domain of the woman. But why does that have to be the case when there's so much fun to be had with both partners hamming it up for the camera? Just choose a song that gets you in the mood, set up that video recorder, and strip the night away.

INDEPENDENT FILM...

You don't actually have to *do it* to make a red-hot home video. Filming each other self-pleasuring yourselves also takes the concept of "home movies" to a hot new level. Each of you needs to take a turn behind the camera—and in front. Watching the videos later will give each of you new insight about what it takes to bring your lover all the way home.

CHOCOLATE PORN

Attention, chocolate lovers: Do some of you really think good chocolate is better than sex? Then it's time to put your money where your money shot is. Bust out all that gooey goodness (by that I mean chocolate syrup, at least for now) and make a film dedicated to chocolate decadence—and deviance. Turn each other into a lovers' sundae, complete with cherry on top. Pour and squirt, lather and smear the chocolate over each other as you film—with your video camera positioned on a tripod and safely away from all the chocolate madness.

NOW YOU KNOW...

There are many safe, fun ways to explore sexuality with technology—and have a great time while you're at it. But even this isn't as kinky as it gets. The next chapter will surely set the kink-o-meter to full power.

Chapter 11

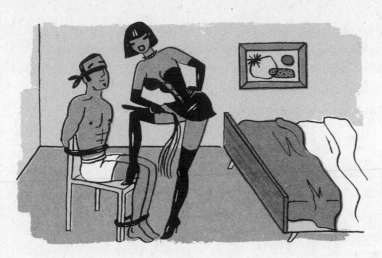

Sometimes Forbidden Is Fabulous

Kinky comes in stages and degrees, spanning from the very mild—like writing your lover's name on your underwear—to the very wild, which we will explore in this chapter.

Consider yourself warned: The activities and suggestions here really do push the concept of kinky to the outer limits, so this chapter is only for those willing to take it almost a step too far. And is there stuff out there even more kinky than what you'll learn in this chapter? You bet. But that's for you and your partner to figure out should you get to the end of this book and still be hot for more.

More so than in previous chapters, open communication, trust, and a sense of humor are key here. So tonight, sit down with your lover and talk it through. Each of you write down your darkest sexual desires—things you've never shared with another living soul. Scenarios, techniques, wishes, you name it. Exchange your lists and really think about what your partner is asking for—what feels like it could still fit into your comfort zone, and what pushes too far. Some of the things you will read will shock you, but keep an open mind. There are surely things on your list that will shock your partner, too.

In this chapter, we'll get into some exciting, sometimes over-the-top possibilities sure to satisfy the most adventurous sexual appetites. From anal sex to strip clubs and sex clubs; from having sex in public to voyeurism; from threesomes and group sex to swinging and more, this is just about as kinky as it gets.

Naughty Nibble

The hottest sexual fantasies are the ones that push you just outside the parameters of what you perceive is your comfort level. Think of it like exercise. You can feel good going at a steady, comfortable clip. But it isn't until you push yourself beyond where you think your limit is that you really hit the zone.

FORBIDDEN FANTASIES

When it comes to fantasy, anything goes. It doesn't matter how it may seem to the world at large. It's not about them. It's only about the two of you, with love, mutual respect, and trust, venturing out on your erotic expedition together. Here are a few fantasies that may go beyond what regular, not-so-kinky folks consider, well, kinky:

The Purple Rose of Porn

Did you ever see the movie *The Purple Rose of Cairo,* in which the male lead of a film actually leaves the screen to be with a woman who's been in the movie theater audience show after show? Now is your chance to be the porn star he can't get enough of. Put on the porn you most like to watch together and leave the room. Now become the leading lady. Does she have red hair or black? Any tattoos? What is she wearing . . . I mean . . . when she's dressed? Copy her outfit, her look, down to her whalebone corset, garter belt, or thigh-highs.

Dress up in your getup and head back to the room where he is. Tell him something like "I know you've been watching me, wondering what it would be like to take me. Well, I've been watching you, too. So let's do it." And take over. Completely. Straddle him and ride him right into the sunset. Or, as another option, copy the action as it's happening on screen. It will be an experience he will never forget.

Extra Credit

She pretends to be a young innocent in high school, a virgin without a clue about the ways of men. He's an older teacher looking for an opportunity to help a bright young student really work for her grades. When she goes to him for "extra help," he gives it to her—you bet he does—as every sex act that can occur between two people does, and in every position imaginable—and right across his desk. Will she make the grade? It's up to him to decide just how much extra work she'll have to do to pass this semester.

We'll Have Nun of That . . .

She's a sister at a struggling church, trying to keep it from closing down. She lives in a terrible, godless neighborhood,

Fun with Fetishes: All Over Your Body

Name a body part and you can be sure someone, somewhere has a fetish for it. Elbows, wrists, head, shoulders, knees, and toes. Here are some of the most common ones:

Breast Fetish

This fetish is not limited to big ones, so ladies, get ready to flaunt whatever you got. Wear different kinds of clothing that show them off, whether that means pushing them together or lifting them high and proud. One day try a sheer shirt—and no bra at all if you're feeling brave. Experiment with this for a full week and see if your guy truly is a breast man.

Foot Fetish

Some people get very turned on playing with or admiring the feet of others. You don't have to take it to extremes to have fun experimenting with foot fetishes, though. Women can draw attention to their feet by having a pedicure and wearing sandals as often as possible. And there are some men who like to have their toenails painted. Are you one of them? If so, ask your partner if she'd be up for giving you a pedicure—complete with a sexy foot massage.

Hand Fetish

I love my man's hands. I watch the way he uses them . . . daily. So when we are intimate, I pay close attention to how he is using them and I get really turned on. Next time your man or woman touches you, pay attention to how they use their hands and see if that enhances your pleasure as well.

Hair—and No Hair—Fetish

Some people are turned on by shaved privates, and some are more turned on when there's hair everywhere. Experiment with this. Try not "grooming" for a while and see if the added friction turns you or your partner on. Then try the reverse: Each of you can shave off *all* your body hair and then make love. Smooth and slick.

where no one goes to church and everyone's out for themselves. But she needs to keep her church alive, and if that means going door-to-door to beg for donations, then that's just what she'll have to do. Because she will do anything—or anyone—to save her church.

Whom she encounters and what they ask of her are up to you, the limits of your own imaginations, and your comfort zones. They are drug lords, prostitutes, thugs, hustlers, and all kinds of lowlifes who won't part with their cash out of the goodness of their hearts. What will be expected of her? How many needs will she need to service—one at a time or for the good of the entire gang? And how far will she really be willing to go? Again, this is all up to you, your imaginations, and, above all else, your boundaries. Have fun!

Traffic Citation

Here's a great one for guys who like to be in power—and one you can play in your own garage. Tell your woman to go down to the garage and sit in the driver's seat of the car until you come for her. [Important: Do *not* turn the car on!] Now slip into the police officer costume you rented earlier in the day and top it off with a pair of dark sunglasses.

Once you're costumed up, head down to the garage and knock on her window with your knuckles or fake nightstick. It really all depends on how sadistic you're feeling. When she unrolls the window, give her the business—and try not to crack up too much. "Do you know how fast you were going . . ." et cetera, et cetera.

Hopefully, she will play along and tell you how sorry she is, but you are not to have any mercy on her. Tell her to get out of the car. Then bend her over the hood, lift up her dress, pull her underwear to the side—not off—and show her what happens to sexy women who break the law in your jurisdiction. . . .

The Carnal Captive

Which one of you decides to be captive or captor is up to you, but the scenario goes something like this: One of you has something the other one, a desperate fugitive on the run, needs. Perhaps it's information, perhaps it's just simply a human hostage the fugitive needs for bargaining. Whatever the case, one of you will be completely dominant in this scenario and the other completely submissive. Before you get into things, be sure you understand the parameters, each other's boundaries, and if a little playful "torture" will become involved here, make darn sure you have your safety word picked and known!

You can start this scenario with your hostage already in custody, or you can actually do the capture as well. Really, it's whatever you, um, desire. Capture your hostage in public in a discreet fashion (you don't want to get arrested here!) or

within the confines of your own home. Take them by surprise and forcefully let them know what's going on and what
will be expected of them. Lead them to your bedroom (or
another room in your home—whatever you want) and instruct them to sit quietly on a chair, on the bed, on the floor.
Then bind them and even gag them if you like. Just not too
tight—remember, this is make-believe. Now, what you want
from them, what will be expected, depends on the fantasy
you devised and agreed upon. You may have some room to
improvise—just be sure you stick to the rules as already out-
lined.

I WANT TO @&#% YOU LIKE AN ANIMAL . . .

Familiar with the song by Nine Inch Nails? Just a wee bit curious about what it means to be @&#%ed this way? So make
believe! Test out your animal magnetism as you pretend to be
animals and make love the way you think your chosen species
would. You could even take it a step further, donning bunny
ears or a cat tail or other accessories reminiscent of the animal you choose. Kinky? Absolutely. Over the
top? No doubt. But this is what it means to
push your limits—to really use your sexual
imagination. And believe it or not, I have
many otherwise well-adjusted clients who
enjoy this kind of play very much.

ON THE SURFACE

Not all anal play means penetration. If you
just want to experiment with the sensitivity
of that area, place a vibrating Bullet or the

> **naughty nibble**
> The anus is actually a
> highly sensitive area,
> rich in nerve endings,
> so it's no wonder so
> many people—whether
> they admit it or not—
> get such a charge from
> buttplay.

tip of a Pocket Rocket at the entrance of your anus, but not inside. As you engage in other activities, you might find it enhances the sensation of what's going on in front and actually makes you more orgasmic.

BACK-DOOR BETTY...

The subject of anal sex always comes up on my radio shows, and mostly from men wanting to take it to the next level with their partners. It's actually a big fantasy for men. Does that mean you should do it? Well, if you're not completely freaked out by it, why not give it a try—with the following parameters firmly in place:

- *Use lots of lube.* I mean, tons. And a water-based lubricant is best.
- *Involve a condom.* Even if you're just entering with a finger, a condom will ease entry and also help keep bacteria at bay.
- *Slow and steady wins the race.* Never force your way into this very delicate area. Not only will it be incredibly uncomfortable for you both, the excess friction could result in unpleasant tears or fissures—his and hers.
- *The bottom is the top.* Meaning, she's in charge of the action here—the speed, the level of penetration, the duration. When she calls it quits, it's over. Period.

Recommended positions include sitting doggie, where he enters from behind but she's folded onto her knees in a crouching position, and missionary, with pillows under her tush to lift her to the right level. Just remember that this is supposed to be a mutual, enjoyable, consensual, sensual activity. But again, if it hurts or is too uncomfortable, it's over.

... AND BOB

Guys, too, can get a lot of pleasure from back-door action. And no, it doesn't mean he's gay if he likes it. He has as many sensitive nerve endings there as she does, and if both partners are comfortable with the idea of it, why not explore it? At the very least, you'll be able to cross it off the list; at best, he'll discover a whole new pleasure zone.

> ### Naughty Nibble
> There is a product called Analease that helps desensitize the tissue around the anus, which makes being entered a little bit easier. (See Resources.)

Just as you would with her, have plenty, I mean plenty, of water-based lube at hand. Start him off on his back and pour some lube over his package—his full package. Now relax him by massaging his shaft and his testicles. Pour on a little more lube and massage down to the perineum. Really press your index and middle fingers into the perineum as you massage, which will indirectly stimulate his prostate. Now massage, massage, massage for at least ten minutes. He should be nice and relaxed by now.

He can move to his tummy or stay on his back—he just needs to bend his legs at the knees to allow access. Place a condom over your finger, or better yet, if you have access to surgical gloves, try that out (you can use more of your fingers at once this way).

Don't just plunge right in. Add more lube, and gently massage his anus with your index finger, pressing lightly first and then adding pressure. Now insert just the very tip of your index finger and wiggle it around in a small circular motion, then out again. Resume the perineum massage with your one hand; reenter him with the fingertip of your other hand, this time making larger circles.

As he gets more and more relaxed and into it, insert your finger a bit deeper and start pulsating it, making a kind of "come hither" motion. You don't have to enter more than a couple of inches in to stimulate the prostate. Just go slow and see if you can bring him to climax this way—it's been known to happen.

Naughty Nibble

Surgical gloves are great when messy things will be happening, but they also make for great props: If your lover's misbehaving, you can always give him or her a light little spanking with them.

MUD MANIA

Have you ever watched mud wrestling— maybe on TV or as part of a movie—and wondered what all the hullabaloo was about? Mud wrestling looks sexy, as it's slippery and slick and oh so dirty . . . and it feels pretty sexy, too. Imagine rolling around with your lover, teased like crazy as you slide up and down and over each other without being able to get a grip. It makes for a lot of fun as foreplay, and it isn't that hard to accomplish. Just keep it outside.

Buy one of those plastic kids' pools and fill it with mud and water (on a day your kids are with your inlaws or other out-of-the-way location). Slip into your bathing suits—or, even better, slip out of your clothing altogether—and wrestle around for a while. You can make love all muddy and nasty, or go savor the sensual steam of a nice hot shower taken together as you help each other get scrubbed clean.

Pleasure Swing

Like the rocking chair in the sex toys chapter, a sex swing guarantees an exciting sexual experience through the motion you derive. Depending on which model you choose, a sex swing can be pricey—sometimes as much as two hundred bucks—but if you love the experience, it's worth the investment.

Once installed, there are countless ways to use it. She can swing in it, suspended just enough to be lowered onto his member. He can swing in it, suspended just enough to graze the tip of her womanhood. What naughty uses will you invent? (See Resources.)

THE PUBLIC EYE

Have you ever had sex in a public place? I don't mean in the privacy of your car—as thin as that privacy is. I mean right out in the open for the world to see, but disguised enough so you keep 'em guessing.

One great place is at the beach. Head out into the surf with your lover and hold on to each other as you rock and kiss. People swimming bob up and down all the time. How will anyone know if you've removed your bathing suits while you're out there? And if anyone figures it out, so what. How would they ever prove it?

Stretch your imagination and see what other options you come up with. Whatever you decide, here's something that may spark an inspiration or two: Imagine the possibilities if she goes out wearing a long skirt with nothing underneath. . . .

WATCH THIS!

Sometimes having an audience when you're having sex is accidental—you didn't realize you'd be visible from the other side of that tree, and so forth. And sometimes it's intentional. Some people, and you may be two of them, really get off on performing for an audience. If this sounds like you, just be sure you're discreet about it and it at least *looks* like an accident.

If you live in an apartment building, do it in front of an open window or on the rooftop—especially effective if you're living in the shortest building in the neighborhood. If you live in the burbs, your backyard, of course, is a natural choice. More-kinky options include having sex in a public bathroom (don't lock the door) or even a janitor's closet. The most obvious choice here is to visit a sex club, go to a swinger's party, and find your way into an orgy. But we'll get into these a little more in just a bit.

STRIP CLUB

Can a woman have a good time at a strip club? Of course she can. Beautiful women, free in their bodies and with their sexuality, can be very inspiring and also arousing—for even the most straight, or straitlaced woman. Of course, this will depend on the kind of strip club you decide to go to. This is going to require a little research on your part. Think "gentlemen's club," not "strip joint," and you should be all right.

It would be exceptionally kinky for the ladies to grab your men and tell them you're heading to a strip club tonight. But no matter how the inspiration strikes, keep your head about it—the both of you. Ladies, leave your jealousy monitor at the door. Gentlemen, behave yourselves, no matter how arousing it is having your lady there with you. Consider your experience at the strip club as foreplay for the action you're going to enjoy once you make it home—if you can hold out that long.

Daring ladies: Buy your man a lap dance. Study the dancer's moves, and see what he responds to and how. Make some mental notes for the next time you play "stripper."

Really daring ladies: Buy your man a lap dance and tell the dancer, step by step, inch by inch, every way you want to see her move around on your man.

Really, *really* daring ladies: Buy yourself a lap dance. Have a little fun with the dancer, who will totally ham it up for you, and be sure to make lots of eye contact with your guy while the dancer gyrates up and down all over you. If you aren't married yet, this last maneuver will probably get you a ring.

FUN TO WATCH

In Thailand, I visited a sex club with my partner and saw several live sex shows. On stage, practically close enough for us to touch, a couple engaged in every sex act you can imagine, with strobe lights flashing and techno music pulsating. Even though all we did was watch, whoa, what a turn-on it was.

You don't have to go to Thailand for this kind of experience. It takes some looking, but you can find shows like this in the States—though probably not as intense. You can appreciate the show as a whole; you can examine every angle, thrust, moan, and groan, and note if anything about it appeals to you as something you want to try. The hottest thing

Naughty Nibble

If you feel like you're just not getting—or giving—enough kinky stimulation from a wooden spoon or other innocent spanking device, it's time to whip out the big guns. I mean whip. Like you'd find in a stable. Or, better yet, a riding crop. Those who really get off on the physical sensation of pain, not just the suggestion of it, swear by props like these— the real thing.

about it is watching something forbidden and violating a taboo. Very, very hot—but definitely not for everyone.

HER LITTLE PET

For a man who craves to be dominated whose partner does not like to dominate: How about calling in a professional domina-trix? His partner gets to stay in the room and watch as her man gets tantalizingly tortured by a woman trained in the fine art of carnal control. She may end up learning a thing or two, or they may both decide together it isn't for them.

Whatever you do, keep the lines of communication wide open—which we'll also stress a bit later on with threesomes and more. Any kind of sex that goes outside the boundaries of your relationship and involves another person has to be talked about in advance and all parties must agree on the rules before, in this instance, the first spanking can occur.

THE NEXT-BEST THING

Are you curious about having a threesome but terrified to actually bring another person into your bed? Go for the next-best thing: fantasy. Although here you can actually add a dose of reality. . . .

You know those nasty 900 numbers, right? The ones

you call to listen to a woman having sex? While you're in the act, dial one up, hit the speakerphone button, and enjoy your third party—live or recorded. It may turn you on, it may crack you up. But either way, you can sample what a threesome may be like and get a little closer to deciding if this is really something you want. (We'll get more into this a bit later on.)

THE GANG'S ALL HERE

You just experienced the safest threesome known to man; now how about an orgy? Have you ever fantasized about what it would be like to have sex with multiple partners all at once? Now here's a way to try it out. You will need: a DVD player, a group-sex DVD, the biggest TV in your home.

Lay down some pillows and blankets in front of the TV and pop in the DVD. While the action heats up on screen, get your partner ready as well, stripping them down, oiling and lubing them up, perhaps even playing with them a little to get them closer to "the mood" as you watch the action unfold. Now jump in . . . I mean, pretend to. Choose a character and imitate everything that person does—to everyone. Your dirty mind will have you transported there in no time, all while keeping your actions—and your body—fairly clean.

Naughty Nibble

Where can you find a professional dominatrix? Many large cities like New York and Los Angeles are crawling with them, if you know where to look. Do a search on Google using the keywords "professional dominatrix," "legal dominatrix clubs," or "legal dominatrix dungeons." Some dungeons list their prices and rules. Some also post photos of the doms available for you to select from. Avoid posting your own ad, however. At least with a legal club, you have some level of protection. Without this filter, you never know whom you're going to end up with.

BUNNY HOP

If the 900-number woman does not satisfy your curiosity and desire, and if you are really determined to experience a threesome, tread with incredible caution. If your third party is a friend, your friendship will never be the same. If it's a stranger—is that really safe? What do you know about this person in terms of diseases or the harboring of *Fatal Attraction* tendencies? If you really must see what it's all about, try a professional. The Moonlight Bunny Ranch in Carson City, Nevada, is a legal brothel that specializes in making fantasies like this one come true. The girls are required to get frequent checkups and screenings, and condoms are always required. That at least takes care of the "physical health" aspect of things. In terms of mental—and relationship—health? There'd better be a lot of dialogue between the two of you leading up to this event. Discuss your concerns and your parameters—what's allowed and what isn't. And be 150 percent sure about it before you do anything at all. (See Resources for contact information.)

YOURS, MINE . . . AND THEIRS

If you feel you'd like to give a threesome a try—with a real live third party—the most important rule is that anything that goes on must have the unconditional consent of all three parties. It's more common to have a threesome involving two women and one man, usually with the women pleasuring each other while the man watches. But not always. Sometimes he's allowed to join in on the action—again, with carefully spelled out restrictions that everyone agrees to ahead of time. Sometimes he's allowed to do only certain acts, like orally pleasuring his wife while the other girl watches—or even orally pleasuring both women, but with no intercourse with the third party. Maybe he's permitted to receive hand stimulation by the third party but can go all the way with his wife. There are so many possibilities, it really comes down to what all parties involved are comfortable allowing and exploring.

The same goes for two men and a woman. Maybe she's allowed to orally service both of them, but allowed to be entered only by her partner. Maybe her partner will allow the third party to penetrate her—with him watching close by, or even with his member in her mouth. While a threesome involving two women and a man usually involves the women servicing each other, this is usually not the case when two men are involved in a threesome with one woman. Most of the time, they share her and leave each other alone. Again, it all depends on your own levels of curiosity and what you're willing to experience and accept.

But whatever you decide, there can be no changes to the action in the heat of the moment; if someone steps out of line, the party's over.

> **Just for Him . . .**
> Hey, she's just not that into you. Okay, she's probably into you, but maybe she's not into sharing you with another woman. So don't push it. Accept that no means no and move on. And keep this in mind: If you can have two ladies, what's to say her fantasy doesn't involve you and another guy? Would you really be willing to try that?

TAKE MY WIFE, PLEASE

Swingers have sex with other people while their partners are present. If your relationship is in trouble, there is no better way to end it than to embark on a quest such as this. Swinging is not something you dabble in—it's a life choice. So don't enter this realm lightly. Talk it over. A lot. You may even try to attend an event—just to watch. Sometimes this is possible for both partners, sometimes only for women. The most important thing if you and your partner do decide that you both are interested in this kind of open sexuality is that you'd better have a strict creed of dos and don'ts lined up before you attend any swingers' gathering.

Most swingers' functions don't allow males to attend alone, and couples are almost always preferred. Swingers' parties or functions are held at private residences, clubs, hotels, resorts, and even cruises. There are also conventions and all kinds of private get-togethers for people who enjoy swinging.

Naughty Nibble

You don't have to look too hard on the Internet to get information on swinging. Do Google searches for "alternative lifestyle conventions," "swingers' clubs," "alternative lifestyle cruises." Don't just go with the first entry that pops up; do your research to find the right group for you both.

IT'S A BACCHANAL, BABY!

The ancients were famous for their appetites, especially when it came to giant feasts of food—and flesh. They loved their orgies, and the concept of getting together in a group to have sex did not fall with Rome. This situation exists from time to time at swingers' functions, but also in more private settings.

HOT POTATO

"Honey, the guys are coming over to watch the game today. Would you mind doling out drinks and snacks—and maybe a few blow jobs while you're at it?" Okay, so this scenario belongs in fantasy and role-play about

99 percent of the time, but for the other 1 percent . . . Well, just as some couples have pushed their personal boundaries to include a third party in their bedroom business, others have explored realms outside of just one other person involved. Is it a fantasy of yours to service your man's friends in front of him, or to have your woman become the main attraction on the buffet table for your friends?

Just like having a threesome or becoming involved in swinging or group sex is something that requires the utmost honesty and crystal-clear communication, so does something like this. Quite possibly, you will not be seeing these friends again, and if things go badly, the only person you may be seeing outside your marriage is a marriage counselor. Remember that a lot can be accomplished in fantasy. If you absolutely must proceed further, please do so with all your wits, um, well-cocked.

NOW YOU KNOW . . .

From mostly innocent to totally insane, from mild to wild, there truly is something for everyone when it comes to kinky. So explore it. Devour it. And enjoy making wonderfully deviant memories together. Just never forget why you got here in the first place—to nurture, savor, and cement the relationship with the one you love above all.

Dennis Hof's World Famous Bunny Ranch
     69 Moonlight Road
     Mound House, NV 89706
     775–246–9901
     888-bunnyranch
     bunnyranch.com
In business since 1955.

PRODUCTS

Adam and Eve
     800–293–4654
     adamandevetoys.com
Toys for women and men, DVDs, and other products.

AdultDVDEmpire.com
DVDs plus adult-movie downloads (pay by the movie or the minute) right to your computer, sex toys, adult novelties, and more.

Babeland
     800–658–9119
     babeland.com
Toys for women and men, DVDs, and more.

Blissbox.com
DVDs plus adult-movie downloads (pay by the movie or even the scene) right to your computer, lingerie, sex toys, and more.

CandidaRoyalle.com
Erotica, porn by women for women, sensual toys by Candida Royalle, pioneer of women's adult erotic movies and author of *How to Tell a Naked Man What to Do*.

Coco de Mer (also in the UK)
    8618 Melrose Avenue
    Los Angeles, CA 90069
    310–652–0311
    cocodemerusa.com
Designer sex toys and lingerie, specialized leather goods, erotic housewares and accessories, erotic books and movies, erotic jewelry, and more.

Come As You Are (Canada)
    701 Queen Street West
    Toronto, Ontario M6J 1E6, Canada
    877–858–3160
    comeasyouare.com
A cooperatively run sex-toy, book, and DVD store.

Forbidden Fruit
    108 East North Loop Blvd.
    Austin, TX 78751
    800–315–2029
    forbiddenfruit.com
Sex toys, costumes, and other adult products, workshops, and more.

Good Vibrations
    800-BUY-VIBE
    goodvibes.com
Sex toys, DVDs and video on demand, books, and more. Several store locations in San Francisco area.

Larry Flynt's Hustler Hollywood
    hustlerhollywood.com
DVDs, books, magazines, sex toys, and more.

Acknowledgments

This book wouldn't even be possible without my husband, Charlie; Carty Talkington, Virginia McAlester, Jennifer Griffin, and Sharon Bowers of the Miller Agency; editor Hallie Falquet of Broadway Books; and the extraordinary Francine LaSala. Thank you so much.

So many instilled in me the confidence and inspiration needed to complete this book. First I want to thank my parents. Little did they know they'd brought a sex therapist into the world, but their support has meant the world to me. Also to my brothers Frank, Lance, and Omar, who have taught me so much about life and relationships, and who love me no matter what, and to Marjorie Bach Walsh, the sister I never had. A big thanks to Tony Cahill, Mark Stahl, Stephen Rice, Mike E., Robert Lyons, Harvey Kalikow, Monica Trinca, Lisa J., Kim P., Lynn Downing, Devon Fischer, JT Unruh, Gary Moon, Ted McIlvenna, Chris Raad, Dr. Bob Schwartz and Leah Schwartz, John Hayden, Gomu, Marc B., C. Sheen, Steve Sanchez, Kevin Antill, David Sack, Dan Theade, JP, Gomez, Nonie Ariate, Beth Walker, Mariska and Blair Nicholson, Michelle Nelson, Ray Davis, and all my wonderful and wild boyfriends and girlfriends who have shared their sexy secrets with me throughout the years (you know who you are). Last but not least, thank you to all the wonderful producers and hosts who have invited me to make so many radio and TV appearances throughout the years. I love you guys.